Studying for Your Midwifery Degree

Siobhan Scanlan and Hilary Walker

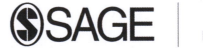

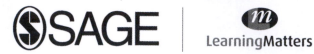

Learning Matters
An imprint of SAGE Publications Ltd
1 Oliver's Yard
55 City Road
London EC1Y 1SP

SAGE Publications Inc.
2455 Teller Road
Thousand Oaks, California 91320

SAGE Publications India Pvt Ltd
B 1/I 1 Mohan Cooperative Industrial Area
Mathura Road
New Delhi 110 044

SAGE Publications Asia-Pacific Pte Ltd
3 Church Street
#10–04 Samsung Hub
Singapore 049483

Editor: Alex Clabburn
Development editor: Richenda Milton-Daws
Production controller: Chris Marke
Project management: Diana Chambers
Marketing manager: Tamara Navaratnam
Cover design: Wendy Scott
Typeset by: Kelly Winter
Printed by Henry Ling Limited at
The Dorset Press, Dorchester, DT1 1HD

Library of Congress Control Number: 2013947936

British Library Cataloguing in Publication data

A catalogue record for this book is available from the British Library

ISBN 978-1-4462-5677-0 (Paperback)
ISBN 978-1-4462-5676-3 (Hardback)

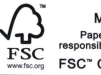

MIX
Paper from
responsible sources
FSC™ C013985
www.fsc.org

Contents

About the authors

Siobhan Scanlan is a clinical midwife in Oxford, a coordinator of a busy delivery suite and a Supervisor of Midwives. She has a PGCE and since 2006 has worked part-time for Oxford Brookes University as an associate lecturer.

Hilary Walker was a tutor in social work at Ruskin College Oxford prior to her retirement. Her previous teaching experience was in social care and child care at Southwark College. She has an extensive background in social work practice, including working as a probation officer, in family centres and as a children and families social worker in a London Borough. She is currently a safeguarding worker for the Methodist Church.

Acknowledgements

We would like to thank the following:

* Richenda Milton-Daws for her consistent support and wise guidance;
* Pete for his sustaining dinners;
* everyone from whom we have learnt – students, colleagues, teachers of midwives and people who use midwifery services;
* each other for mutual learning.

Introduction

This book is written for students undertaking pre-registration courses in midwifery. Its main purpose is to support you in your studies by identifying the academic skills that must be demonstrated in an undergraduate degree and explaining how this relates to learning to become a midwife. Because it makes these connections, it may also be of use to postgraduate midwifery students.

Most people reading this will have been selected for a place on a midwifery course or already be studying. When you examine the programme ahead of you in more detail you will find that it has been developed and organised in order to meet general requirements laid down by the Quality Assurance Agency for Higher Education (QAA), the body with responsibility for assuring the quality of higher education courses in universities and colleges. Although each course is organised in a different way, universities must ensure that students studying on a bachelor degree with honours will have achieved what is set out in this framework by the end of the programme. Because learning happens in stages, each building on earlier understanding, these requirements are organised in three levels known as 4, 5 and 6. For full-time students these will be equivalent to the three years of the degree. For part-time students this will depend on the course.

Requirements at each level specify what students must be able to do and demonstrate academically at each level of the programme. A bachelor degree with honours must provide the opportunity for students to achieve this through teaching, learning and assessment. Of course, a degree in chemistry or French will look different from a degree in midwifery, but the same broad academic requirements must be met.

In addition to the broad requirements set by the QAA, undergraduate degrees in midwifery must also meet requirements laid down in the Nursing and Midwifery Council's *Standards for pre-registration midwifery education* (NMC, 2009).

Achieving a degree in midwifery is about being able to practise, but equally about being able to demonstrate academic capabilities and skills at undergraduate degree level. It is both a licence to practise as a professional midwife and an academic qualification. Midwifery is an applied academic subject so practice is an essential and core element of learning, and you will be required to spend at least half of the course undertaking learning on placement. By the end of the course you must have met both the academic and practice standards, and you will find that these two aspects are consistently and constantly interconnected. You will be required to make links between what you learn in university and the world of midwifery, and think about, understand, critically analyse and reflect on your practice while in placement using academic learning.

However, these requirements indicate what you must be able to do by the end of your course rather than the stages along the way. In contrast, as discussed above, the general requirements for an undergraduate honours degree set out what students should achieve at each level. Because learning is cumulative, you need to have a sound grasp of lower-level academic skills in order to build towards the higher ones. Students can sometimes struggle later in their studies if they have not thoroughly developed foundation skills.

This book therefore takes a staged approach and is organised in three parts – each one relating to a different academic level. Hence chapters in Part One will be concerned with skills from Level 4, those in Part Two with skills from Level 5 and those in Part Three from Level 6. In each part of the book the key academic requirements at that level are explored. Every chapter indicates the specific requirements to which it relates. On your course, in university and on placement, this division will not be as clear. However, separating them out should help you to appreciate the skills you are using and enhancing.

The four chapters in Part One cover the basic foundation academic skills. The first explores beginning your degree course and the particular characteristics of studying for midwifery, before discussing different approaches to learning. In Chapter 2 we focus on the underlying principles and concepts in midwifery with particular emphasis on the values. In Chapter 3 the relationship between theory and midwifery practice is considered, while in Chapter 4 the ingredients of academic writing are covered.

This theme is developed in Part Two, as Chapter 5 looks at more complex skills of critical analysis and understanding. Chapter 6 focuses on learning in practice and how to make connections between your university studies and your experiences and practice on placement. In Chapter 7 we explore what is meant by the reflective midwife practitioner and ways in which this approach can be enhanced. The final chapter of Part Two is the first of two looking at research. At this level the focus is on understanding and using research.

Part Three begins with the second research chapter, which explains how research can be subject to critical evaluation. In Chapter 10 we return to thinking about learning and focus on becoming an autonomous learner. The final two chapters both consider the complexity of midwifery. In Chapter 11 we consider the academic purposes of the dissertation or project and some helpful ways of approaching this important and complex piece of work. In Chapter 12 the complicated and contradictory nature of practice is analysed, and the thinking and reflective skills and strategies for midwives working in this context are discussed.

There is a glossary of terms at the end of the book that provides an interpretation of some of the terminology in the context of the subject of the book. Glossary terms are in bold in the first instance that they appear.

In order to illustrate the development of learning through the degree we will follow the studying experiences of three midwifery students. Nazneen has joined her course with A-level qualifications and some relevant experience. Paul, a mature student, has a wide range of experiences and has met the academic entrance requirements. Linda has previously qualified and worked as a nurse and now wishes to retrain and specialise in midwifery. You will see the challenges they face and how they are able to develop into effective learners who are able to move into the role of a qualified midwife.

Each chapter could be read on its own; however, you will probably find it most helpful to use the entire book. This is, first, because it will help you to follow the learning journeys of the three midwifery students throughout the book and, second, because interconnections are made between chapters. In many chapters you will find guidance on how to approach a particular academic skill. This is based on observations from our own experience as tutors and what we have learnt from students and research studies into what helps students learn. Within each chapter you will find examples and activities to support you with the development of the relevant skills. However, the book is not a substitute for fully participating in all the learning activities on your course. Rather, its purpose is to be complementary to your university learning and to help you make the most of it. You should always make sure you are clear about the assessment requirements and regulations on your particular programme.

During our work in teaching and midwifery we have come across a wide range of students. Nearly all students find some aspect of their academic work a challenge – sometimes because their interest is more on doing midwifery. One reason for writing this book was to make clear that midwifery cannot be practised well without good, clear, analytic thinking. Another was to provide students with some materials that would better enable them to face and overcome the challenges. We hope it has succeeded. Good luck in your studies.

Part One

Chapter 1
Beginning your midwifery education

Chapter aims

After reading this chapter you will be able to:

- understand what will be expected of you when studying for the degree in midwifery;
- appreciate the particular characteristics of midwifery education;
- identify what knowledge, skills and experience you bring to the course;
- discover some effective ways for you to study, learn and develop.

Introduction

The purpose of this chapter is to help you to think about some important aspects of studying for a midwifery degree and what you will need to consider when embarking on your studies. It will provide you with some ways of approaching the challenge of studying in a positive and constructive way.

The degree in midwifery

Studying for any undergraduate degree is a demanding undertaking. For students of midwifery there are particular features and requirements that provide added challenges. In the first part of this chapter we will explore these and highlight the implications for you. The degree in midwifery enables you to develop an understanding of the art and science of midwifery, and the concepts of lifelong learning.

A range of midwifery settings

The qualification you receive at the end of your education enables you to practise autonomously across different settings of the maternity services – for example, in the community, midwifery-led units, birth centres and hospitals. You will gain an appreciation of the importance of working in a multidisciplinary team with a range of other professionals, including obstetricians, health visitors, social workers, physiotherapists and pharmacists (DH, 2007). You should also have the opportunity to practise with midwives who have a specialised area of work within public health, such as working with vulnerable groups or prenatal advice clinics. During your practice placements you will develop greater knowledge, skills and understanding in these different settings. When studying for your degree you will need to think broadly about the very wide range of services, agencies and service users that are a part of contemporary midwifery practice. The examples in this book have been drawn from different contexts to assist with this.

Incorporating perspectives of women and families

The participation and involvement of people who use the services of midwives has become a key issue in current midwifery policy, practice, research and education. Women who use midwifery services may be involved in the selection of students, teaching and assessment on your course, and in its design, delivery and evaluation (NMC, 2013a). When studying on a midwifery degree, thinking deeply about and actively taking into consideration the experiences and perspectives of women and families who use the maternity services are essential. As Professor Paul Lewis (2011, p6) argues, '*What does this mean for the woman in our care?*' *is the question we should constantly ask ourselves.* This means that you will have to give careful attention to the various ways of expanding your understanding of these perspectives.

There are several ways in which you can learn more about the views of women and families. First, you could access documents produced by campaigning groups such as National Childbirth Trust (NCT) and the Association for Improvements in the Maternity Services (AIMS). Second, it is, of course, expected that student midwives will listen actively to the women they are caring for on placement to learn more about their lives and experiences. Third, there is a body of literature that presents research into the views and voices of women who use services (NPEU, 2007; RCM, 2008a; Redshaw and Heikka, 2010; Singh and Newburn, 2000).

It is important to bring this understanding of experiences, thoughts and feelings of women and their families into your academic essays and assignments. This is one of the challenges of the degree in midwifery – to be able to integrate – or blend – academic ideas and personal and professional perspectives. However, it is essential as it is part of learning to practise midwifery in a way that is respectful of the lives of the women who use the services. This will be a theme throughout the book.

Learning in practice at an early stage

Within the first few weeks of your degree, you will be shadowing a midwife and observing and working alongside her. This will give you the opportunity of applying what you have been taught in university. This could include physically examining women in a clinical setting, taking blood, examining sutures in the home setting or even attending a birth in a hospital or a community environment. This is the beginning of your learning in practice, which will run alongside your university-based studies. Throughout your course it is important that you continue to develop and connect academic and practice learning.

About half of your degree course will be spent undertaking learning in practice in a hospital or community setting. Some students relish this opportunity to 'get into the real world' and be 'hands on'. It may be tempting to see the two aspects of learning – university and practice – as separate. But it is essential that you appreciate the connection between the two and develop the ability to think about one in relation to the other. Students can find their first experience of practice different from their expectations and sometimes, initially, daunting (Barkley, 2011; Clarke, 2011). However, by using your skills of observation, listening and asking appropriate questions you can soon learn to understand the way in which midwives work and how you can best make use of this experience.

Midwifery is based on a set of ethical values

From its formal beginnings midwifery has paid close attention to its values – what is regarded as important or valuable. It has been understood that the decisions and actions of midwives, and how they go about their work, can have potential for benefit or for harm. All student midwives must learn about and be able to demonstrate these values. The Nursing and Midwifery Council (NMC) regulates professional practice in the UK with the overall aim of safeguarding the health and well-being of the public. All qualified midwives must register with the NMC and submit their 'Notification of Intention to Practise' form before they can practise as a midwife. The NMC produces standards for practising midwives in the *Midwives rules and standards* (NMC, 2012) and in a code (NMC, 2008), which sets out required core values of professional midwives and nurses; these will be discussed later in the book. When you start the course you will be given a copy of the publication *Guidance on professional conduct for nursing and midwifery students* (NMC, 2010), which can be downloaded from the NMC website. From the beginning of your studies you will be learning how abstract concepts such as values and ethical principles are relevant to practice; this will be discussed further in Chapter 2.

In order to set the scene for your studies, we have introduced the degree in midwifery, explored some important aspects and highlighted some of its complexities. With this in mind, in the rest of the chapter we will consider some helpful ways of getting down to studying.

Studying for your degree in midwifery

In this section we will consider some important things to think about before you start studying, such as your own background, how to use previous experience, how learning will challenge you and using the help of others.

About you

Some of you may bring to your course a great deal of experience of life and work, together with previous knowledge and useful, relevant skills – so you will have plenty to build on and lots to contribute to other people's learning. However, there may be aspects of studying with which you may not be familiar. Others may have some recent experience of studying but limited experience of midwifery issues. This activity is designed to help you to become more self-aware of what you bring with you to the course.

Activity 1.1   *Reflection*

What I bring to my degree in midwifery

Try to take a step back and think about yourself – and answer the questions set out below.

- What experience, knowledge and skills do you bring to your studies?
- What aspects of the course do you feel fairly comfortable about tackling?
- What aspects of the course might be a real challenge for you?

Record your answers to these questions and note the date.

Below are answers from three midwifery students, Nazneen, Paul and Linda, who we will be following through their studies.

Nazneen Khan (19 years) wrote:
- *In my gap year I have looked for employment that would help me with clinical and practical caring skills. I worked as a health care assistant for three months in a residential facility for the elderly and then was successful in obtaining a post as a support worker in a busy maternity hospital. I feel confident this experience will help me feel more comfortable in clinical environments when I start my midwifery course. I am also continuing with some volunteer work at a local family centre where a national parenting charity organises a peer-support group.*
- *I was pleased to achieve good results in my A levels and feel this will be a positive foundation for the academic side of the degree course. Speaking Urdu and Punjabi has been more than helpful in my care work, and I think it will be an advantage for me as a student midwife.*
- *Does it matter if you don't have children of your own? This seems to be an important question for women when they meet midwives and support staff for the first time. I feel that I have lots of life experience and that I am mature for my age – but will I be perceived as 'too young' by some of the client group?*

Paul O'Connor (39 years) wrote:
- *When I left school I was in youth work for a few years and then became an auxiliary in an acute admissions ward in a psychiatric hospital. Eight years ago I trained in craniosacral therapy and moved to France to be near my wife's family. My communication and listening skills are good, and I can adapt to changing circumstances and be creative with problem solving.*

- *Having my own children and working with parents and families as a therapist has given me the confidence to approach midwifery education. I've really enjoyed the access course and feel ready for the research and writing side of things.*
- *There are more men in midwifery now, with great role models in the profession. But some women and families will prefer to be cared for by a woman: that might be hard for me. Being an independent practitioner as a midwife has many attractions, but obviously the hospital education will involve me being part of a very large team – will I be able to slot into this easily again?*

Linda Grantham (33 years) wrote:

- *Working as an adult nurse has been fulfilling, but I have been interested in working more closely with mothers and children for a long time. Since having my own children I have been drawn more and more to midwifery and I have been doing organisational work for the breast milk donor service in my area ever since I was on maternity leave. I think I would like to help mothers at higher risk, or work in public health or maybe even neonatal intensive care – but I want to keep all my options open.*
- *I'm a good juggler and I can delegate and organise my own time when it is busy. This will help me balance college work and home – but I know it will still be demanding trying to get assignments done and fitting in the practice hours.*
- *Going back to college as a qualified nurse might be a challenge as I've not done much studying since qualifying as a nurse. I am also wondering what it will be like being a 'learner' again in clinical settings – I need to work out some strategies on how to cope with this one.*

During the course you should, with the help of your tutors, be keeping a record, unique to you, of your progress as a learner throughout your course. This is sometimes known as a **Personal Development Plan** (PDP), but it might also be called a portfolio, and you may find that your college has its own particular format for your PDP. Your answers to the questions in Activity 1.1 could be helpful in identifying the areas in which you feel strong and the areas you feel you need to develop at the beginning of your course. It may also assist you in setting some goals or targets for your learning. Revisiting these during the course and reviewing how much progress you have made will help you to become a self-managing and reflective learner.

Using your experience

From the answers given by the students above it is clear that groups can be very diverse. You will be studying with people from a range of backgrounds and cultures, and with a variety of experiences, and you have the opportunity to learn a lot from them. But the diversity within a group may also be a challenge as you come across people with different perspectives and views on life from yours. Moreover, what you learn on the course may also disquiet you. Although your life and work experience will be valued in group discussions and tutorials, you will also find that your ideas and assumptions concerning such experiences will be challenged by tutors and other students. You will be introduced to new ideas and different ways of thinking that may undermine what you have taken for granted and unsettle you both personally and professionally.

Research summary

David Howard (2002), Pam Green Lister (2000) and Rosalind Edwards (1993) draw on research that clearly highlights the huge impact of this challenge. The experiences described by students included:

- feeling deskilled when they looked back at their previous practice in the light of new knowledge;
- experiencing self-doubt about their ability;
- needing to 'unlearn' some dearly held ideas and ways of doing things;
- some tension with family and friends when the students' ideas and understanding changed and developed.

Case study: Nazneen's learning challenge

Nazneen has recently worked with families on a maternity ward and has some experience of being with mothers and babies from within her own family. In the university teaching on social policy, research into the difficulties of bringing up children in poverty (Ghate and Hazel, 2003) is discussed. Nazneen begins to think about some judgemental assumptions she has made about families where breastfeeding and healthy lifestyles were not a priority. This makes her feel uncomfortable about herself, as she had always thought she was understanding and respectful of others' viewpoints. Now she sees that she had not really considered what the day-to-day lives of some families were like.

Staff teaching on midwifery courses understand that students such as Nazneen and those in the research studies are likely to be challenged during the course and will provide safe ways for them to examine their thoughts and feelings, together with tutorial support. It is important for students to recognise that openness to looking at issues in different ways and having their ideas questioned will assist them in effective learning. The following activity will help you with this.

Activity 1.2   *Critical thinking*

Responding to being challenged

Think about how you respond when your ideas are challenged. Try to answer honestly. Do you:

- become defensive about your ideas?
- feel hurt and angry that you haven't been listened to?
- interrupt and argue back before the challenger has had a chance to explain their position?

continued . . . •••

- agree with the challenge to avoid conflict?
- find it very easy to look at an issue from a different viewpoint?
- find it difficult to put the arguments to defend your position?
- take some time to think about the other person's point?
- weigh up the arguments for and against the other person's ideas?
- try to identify the reasons for holding your viewpoint?
- explore why the reasons for holding the viewpoint are important to you?

In the activity above, you will see that answering 'yes' to the questions at the top of the list indicate reluctance to have ideas questioned and tested, while answering 'yes' to those at the bottom suggest a more open-minded and thoughtful approach. When you consider your answers you might think about whether they indicate that you will find being challenged difficult and whether this could be an obstacle to your learning. Some of the activities later in the book, especially in Chapter 7, will provide you with more opportunities to constructively and reflectively think about your life and any previous employment experiences.

Using others to help you learn

It can be helpful to have a 'critical friend' to support you when having your ideas and experiences questioned. A critical friend is someone: who likes and respects you; who is happy to be a sounding board for your thoughts and ideas; who helps you to be self-questioning; who will be comfortable and confident to challenge you; and with whom you feel safe to explore ideas (Redmond, 2006).

Case study: Linda and Maggie

Linda's friend Maggie was starting the three-year midwifery degree at the same time as Linda began her post-registration course. They had often talked about their shared interest in supporting women in giving birth and found they had some ideas in common but also sometimes quite different perspectives on childbirth that they enjoyed discussing. When they started their courses they developed their 'critical friendship' and through this examined the issues they faced and the new thinking to which they were exposed. They learnt how to challenge each other sensitively and with care – and both Linda and Maggie knew that they had become more thoughtful through their regular discussions.

Sometimes students find support groups and online forums very helpful to their development through the course. This can especially be the case when students have something particular in common, such as discrimination because of sexuality or race either in the university or on placement. Sharing experiences and talking them through in a safe setting outside the classroom can provide support, encouragement and ways to take issues forward.

> ### Case study: Support group – The Association of Radical Midwives (ARM)
>
> *Paul had attended a weekend conference of ARM as he thought it would help him prepare for his midwifery degree. Set up in the 1970s by midwives who were frustrated by the increasing medicalisation and intervention in maternity care at the time, ARM is a campaigning support group whose aim is to share ideas, skills and information with colleagues and clients and to improve midwifery continuity and maternity care. It holds an annual meeting on a particular topic relating to supporting normal birth. Paul felt very welcomed by the group, and had the opportunity to join some informative sessions on aspects of care in labour and breastfeeding support and the chance to meet some interested and committed midwives and students. Some students he had met were planning to attend the Royal College of Midwives (RCM) Student Conference later in the year, and Paul was pleased to make arrangements with his new contacts to go with them. They were keen to share their experiences of university and placement and encouraged him to join the online forums of ARM and Studentmidwife.net.*

How we learn: surface and deep approaches

Having explored some aspects of the midwifery degree, we will now consider different **approaches to learning**. Biggs and Tang (2011), Entwistle et al. (2001) and Coffield (2009) draw a distinction between surface and **deep** approaches to learning. In a surface approach to learning the student wants to get the task over and done, with as little effort as possible, to meet the requirements of the course. Students taking this approach tend to:

- focus on selected facts rather than developing a full understanding;
- list points rather than developing arguments;
- avoid reading beyond the classroom notes and handouts to enhance their appreciation;
- pad out assignments;
- focus on the signs of learning – words used and isolated fact – rather than thinking about meanings and relationships.

In contrast, a deep approach to learning involves:

- becoming actively interested in the content of the course;
- becoming aware of your understanding developing while learning;
- focusing on the underlying meaning of ideas, themes and principles;
- trying to appreciate the relationship between ideas and previous knowledge;
- checking evidence and relating it to conclusions;
- thinking abstractly;
- aiming to think deeply:
- learning from your mistakes.

Entwistle et al. (2001) and Coffield (2009) add a third approach, which they call a **strategic** approach to learning. Learners with this approach:

- aim to achieve the highest goals;
- manage their time and effort effectively;
- find the right conditions and materials for studying;
- monitor the effectiveness of their ways of studying;
- are alert to the assessment requirements of the course;
- gear their work to the perceived preferences of tutors.

Biggs and Tang (2011) and Moon (2005, 2008) argue that a deep approach to learning is essential for students to make progress on degree courses. Entwistle et al. (2001) and Race (2010) add that the focus on organising study and self-monitoring in the strategic approach is also fundamental to successful study.

Activity 1.3   *Reflection*

Your learning approach

Consider whether you tend to take a surface or a deep approach to learning and which aspects of the strategic approach could be applied to you.

Your answer might give you a sense of how you could develop your learning. If, as you progress through the course, you rely on a surface approach to your studies, you will have difficulty with the academic thinking requirements. It is important to note that these approaches are not set in stone or essential parts of your make-up, and you have the potential to change and develop. The teaching, assignments, learning experiences and student support on your degree course will assist you with this. The examples and activities in this book are designed to enable you to develop a deep approach to learning.

Case study: Paul's learning approach

Paul is at risk of taking a surface approach to some aspects of his learning. He starts the course by seeing it as a means to gaining a qualification and feels he knows a great deal about normal midwifery already. He is not seeing the course as an opportunity to deepen his understanding of wider aspects of midwifery, and he wants to focus on 'getting through'. His tutors will be challenging him to move beyond those areas and approaches with which he is familiar – out of his 'comfort zone'.

Biggs and Tang (2011), Race (2010) and Moon (2008) point out that students learn best when they:

- know where they should be going and what they are aiming for;
- are motivated to get there;
- have confidence in their ability to reach their goals;
- feel free to focus deeply on the task;

- have ownership of their learning or '**self-efficacy**';
- can work in partnership with tutors and other students.

Your studying will proceed more smoothly if you try to ensure these factors are in place for you. Understanding how you go about studying, being aware of yourself as a learner and monitoring your own development are important as you move through the course. Moon (2008) and Coffield (2009) discuss how awareness of your own learning can support and encourage its development. This idea of 'metacognition' will be discussed further in Chapter 7 and in greater depth in Chapter 10.

Getting down to studying

In this last part of the chapter we will explore some hints and tips for effective study.

Organising yourself

To study successfully good organisation is essential and should avoid wasting time. It can ensure that you use your time effectively and are able to keep to the course deadlines.

Organising yourself

This is what one midwifery student said about organising yourself.

- *Create a study space for yourself at home: I quickly found that folders, books and journals appeared to breed . . . your own desk, bookshelf, filing cabinet and laptop can bring logic and harmony to your mind and home.*
- *Learn how to say 'no' to unreasonable demands from friends and family; know when you need to make time to have fun.*
- *Use your study days wisely: stay focused and plan ahead so you can make the most of valuable time.*
- *Learn how to use the library: do this as soon as you can if you want to produce work which meets the rigorous standards of your course.*
(Common, 2007)

Here are some tips that students we have taught have found helpful.

Where, when and how to study

- Different people study in different ways. Some people need absolute quiet, and some people like to listen to music. Some like to study late in the evening; some prefer to study early in the morning. Some adults like to study while their children are doing their homework – others don't. You need to work out what is best for you.
- Find a space where you can study with reasonable peace and quiet – think about lighting, heating, comfort and potential distractions. Negotiate with other people in your home so that the space you choose is respected.

- Studying effectively for a few hours and taking regular breaks is generally more productive than slogging away unproductively for hours and hours. Some people find it best to study for 30 minutes and take a 5- or 10-minute break before returning to the task.
- Taking a short walk or some other form of exercise, rather than sitting, frustrated and unable to understand, can be a positive benefit.
- It will reinforce your learning if you read your notes after a teaching session before filing them away.
- Be meticulous with your recording of notes – date each piece and mark the name of the lecturer/tutor involved.
- Make sure you find time to relax.
- Reward yourself for keeping to your schedule.

Keeping papers, books and electronic files in a systematic way

- You may be surprised by the number of books, papers and computer files and folders you collect over three or four years of study. It is really important to be organised from the start. This will save you time later.
- Find a space for your books and papers. This needs to be a place where they will be safe and organised, and where you will easily to be able to find what you need. Later in the course you will need to go back to notes and handouts from your first year. You will get very annoyed with yourself if you can't find them.
- Develop good electronic folder systems and organisation of useful web pages. Always back up your computer files.
- Equip yourself with folders, files, sticky notes of various colours, paper and highlighter pens. File dividers can be helpful.
- Always keep a note of the source of your notes and file your notes away.
- As you go along try out different systems of organising your growing amount of material.

Time management and making the best use of the time you have for study

It may be difficult to find as much time as you would like to spend on your studies so making the best use of your time will be very important.

- Each term, be aware of the deadlines you have to meet and work towards them. Note the deadlines in your diary and on your computer or mobile phone.
- Draw up a weekly schedule of goals you need to achieve in the light of the deadlines you have to meet.
- Try to plan to finalise your work a few days before the hand-in date so you are prepared for last-minute crises (such as computer crashes, illness and family crises).
- Prioritise your work carefully – always start with the most important work. If you are unsure about which work is top priority, discuss it with your tutor.
- Avoid interruptions if you possibly can.
- Negotiate your study time with your family.
- If you have some small chunks of time, use them productively for tasks you can achieve within that space.

- If you are very tired, but need to use the time you have set aside, carry out tasks that are not too demanding and save the more difficult tasks for when you are fresh and alert.
- Keep a list of tasks, and when one is complete, tick it off. This will give you a great sense of achievement.

Looking after yourself

Because the course will be demanding in lots of ways, it is really important to get into good habits of taking care of yourself both physically and emotionally.

Activity 1.4	*Reflection*

Looking after yourself

Make a list of the steps you can take to look after yourself so you can get the most out of the course.

In your answers you might have identified the following.

- Eat healthily.
- Aim to get sufficient sleep.
- Deal with stress constructively: if you are in a state of anxious stress and physically tense, resources are taken away from the brain. Short, brisk exercise can help you shift from this. If you exercise outside, you can benefit from the daylight.
- Take time for yourself and aim to get the study/life balance right.
- Learn some relaxation techniques.
- Use tutorial support to explore issues that are troubling you.
- Access the student support services.
- Have confidence in your ability to learn even if you get stuck and encounter obstacles.

Developing the habit of reading

In order to manage the course successfully you will need to read widely and effectively. One way to build the habit is to read novels or less academic books that deal with issues of relevance to midwifery (some examples are provided at the end of the chapter). To read effectively, select your reading material with care, and learn to skim-read and focus your best energy and attention on the chapters or passages that are relevant to you. Using highlighting and sticky notes will ensure you can easily find the passages to which you will need to return.

Using the internet with care

Using the internet for your studies gives you exciting opportunities to access materials for study such as e-books, journal articles, government reports, policy documents, research and statistics. Being able to access information easily can be helpful to your learning; however, carrying out searches for material needs to be done with care. The internet gives freedom to people to communicate with others via their web pages. However, this also means that extreme and minority views can be widely circulated. Books and journals will have been subjected to review and assessment by editors, but some websites, such as Wikipedia, may not have been through any academic external scrutiny. Google and other search engines may offer unfiltered and unreferenced reading that is too basic (Reisz, 2008). So when you are considering material you need to think about its validity – for example, who has produced the ideas and why. There are websites produced by groups of men who have experienced domestic abuse. However, statistics tell us that it is mostly women who experience serious domestic abuse. So, while the websites can express a valid minority viewpoint, any information used from them needs to be put into context within your essay or assignment.

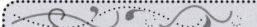

Chapter summary

This chapter has introduced what is required to study for a degree in midwifery and the particular challenges of these courses, and it has highlighted some important issues that students need to take into account during their studies. It has given particular attention to the value of the experiences students bring to the course but also how you need to be open to challenge. Some ways of being supported have been identified. Finally, some helpful ideas for studying have been suggested.

By exploring some of the challenges of the degree in midwifery, this chapter risks alarming and daunting some students. We hope that is not the case and that instead it has captured your interest and excited you about the journey to becoming a qualified midwife. At times you will feel tired and frustrated, but more often you will enjoy learning and developing your understanding, becoming more able to explore ideas, concepts and theories, and really coming to appreciate the joy of studying for your degree in midwifery.

Further reading

Study skills textbooks

Cottrell, S (2013) *The study skills handbook* (4th edition). Basingstoke: Palgrave Macmillan.

Hutchfield, K and Standing, M (2012) *Succeeding in essays, exams and OSCEs for nursing students*. Exeter: Learning Matters.

Northedge, A (2005) *The good study guide*. Buckingham: The Open University.

Scullion, P A and Guest, D A (2007) *Study skills for nursing and midwifery students*. Maidenhead: Open University Press.

These books provide detailed and very helpful advice for studying.

Lee, K and Busby, A (2010) Going to university: hints and tips for new midwifery students. *British Journal of Midwifery*, 8 (10): 669–71.

A very useful article for midwifery students beginning their course.

Personal development planning

Cottrell, S (2010) *Skills for success* (2nd edition). Basingstoke: Palgrave Macmillan.

This very accessible book provides detailed advice about – and helpful activities for – personal development planning.

Reading to help you find out more about midwifery

Flint, C (1986) *Sensitive midwifery*. Oxford: Heinemann.

Although written some time ago, it contains useful thinking about practising women-centred midwifery.

Mander, R and Fleming, V (eds) (2009) *Becoming a midwife* Abingdon: Routledge.

An edited collection of chapters covering a range of midwifery settings and stages in pregnancy narrated by midwives.

Symonds, A and Hunt, S (1994) *The social meaning of midwifery*. Basingstoke: Palgrave Macmillan.

An observational study of labour-ward culture that, although dated, still raises important issues, such as the relationship between women as childbirth professionals and women as mothers.

Novels relevant to midwifery

Below are a few examples of novels on topics relevant to midwifery.

Bohjalian, C (1998) *Midwives* New York: Vintage books.

An American independent midwife responds to a dramatic emergency during a rural home birth and then must deal with the consequences.

Cushman, K (1996) *The midwife's apprentice* New York: Clarion Books.

Although written for older children/adolescents, this is an interesting read for adults. The story is about an orphan girl taken on by a reluctant midwife in mediaeval England.

Doyle, R (1997) *The woman who walked into doors*. London: Vintage.

Set in contemporary Dublin, this story describes how domestic abuse (graphically detailed) gradually erodes dignity, self-esteem and hope, although the central character, Paula, eventually triumphs

Dunmore, H (2003) *Mourning Ruby*. London: Penguin.

A woman's grief following the death of her young child

Emecheta, B (1994) *In the ditch*. Oxford: Heinemann.

A lone Nigerian woman copes with pregnancy and motherhood in London.

Levy, A (2009*) Small Island*. London: Headline Review.

This story of crossed lives and confusions moves between the Second World War and post-war life for the Caribbean and white British characters. The birth scene is sad, funny and unforgettable.

Perkins Gilman, C (2009) *The yellow wallpaper and selected writings*. London: Virago Press.

Written by an eminent American feminist at the turn of the twentieth century, this eerie tale describes how a woman is confined to her bed after childbirth and ordered to stop writing for the sake of her 'nerves' (common advice at the time for creative women acting abnormally). Includes *The unnatural mother*, the story of a woman who made the ultimate sacrifice.

Prager, E (1993) *A visit from the foot binder*. London: Vintage.

An insight into how mothers can contemplate inflicting what seems to be a horrific act on their daughters.

Thompson, Flora (2008) *Lark Rise to Candleford*. London: Penguin Classics.

Beautiful tale of a young girl growing up in Victorian Oxfordshire. It describes birth and community support, and includes one of the loveliest quotes on midwifery in literature.

Useful websites

General websites

Association of Radical Midwives	www.midwifery.org.uk
Cochrane Database of Systematic Reviews	www.cochrane.org
Nursing and Midwifery Council	www.nmc-uk.org
Royal College of Midwives	www.rcm.org.uk
Student midwives	www.studentmidwife.net

Websites on study skills

There are many websites devoted to skills for study. There are risks in accessing these. Their specific guidance (e.g. on referencing or essay construction) may differ from those of the university where you are studying, or be targeted at a different academic level. It may therefore be best to use the guidance provided on your course and use websites only for very general advice. Given that proviso, the following websites may be useful.

www2.open.ac.uk/students/skillsforstudy

www.palgrave.com/skills4study/studyskills

Chapter 2
Understanding and using concepts and principles
Values and midwifery

This chapter will help you to meet the Quality Assurance Agency for Higher Education (QAA, 2008) requirement that students studying at Level 4 are able to:

- demonstrate knowledge of the underlying concepts and principles associated with their area(s) of study, and an ability to evaluate and interpret these within the context of that area of study.

NMC Standards for Pre-registration Midwifery Education

This chapter will address the following competencies:

Domain: Professional and ethical practice
Practise in a way which respects, promotes and supports individuals' rights, interests, preferences, beliefs and cultures.

Maintain confidentiality of information.

Chapter aims

After reading this chapter you should be able to:

- understand concept and principle as academic terms;
- identify significant concepts used in midwifery;
- appreciate the main principles of midwifery;
- recognise how values are integral to midwifery.

Introduction

The purpose of this chapter is to explore some major concepts and principles that provide the foundation for midwifery thinking. It aims to provide ways of helping you to grasp what these are and appreciate their relevance.

Understanding concepts and principles

Without a good understanding of what concepts and principles are, and how they are used, it is difficult to take a deep approach to your learning and move on to other stages of the degree. It will be of benefit to you later to invest time now in order to achieve a sound appreciation of them. In order to support you with this, we will explore the meaning of both concepts and principles before considering some examples, using activities to embed your understanding.

First, it is worth considering what it means to really understand an issue. Biggs and Tang (2011) argue that one level of understanding occurs when people are able to explain something or answer questions on it. This is known as declarative or propositional knowledge. But real understanding changes the way people perceive the world, and as a result they do things differently – this is known as functioning understanding. Over the course of the degree your level of knowledge and appreciation of issues should develop and deepen. As this happens, you should find your understanding increases and you are able to use your knowledge to decide why, how and in which order to do things and solve problems. In midwifery this means using your understanding to guide how you go about your practice. In this chapter we are concerned mostly with declarative or propositional knowledge – knowing about things – but because both midwifery and midwifery education is about change and transformation we may also touch upon deeper understandings.

We will first explore the notion of concepts and identify some important concepts in midwifery before exploring some ways of learning to grasp them.

Concepts

A concept has been defined as *a mental representation of a group of items which are similar in some way* (Cottrell, 2013, p295). Alternatively *The Oxford Dictionary of English* (second edition) (2008) defines a concept as *an abstract idea*. So considering a concept means thinking in an abstract and general way – moving beyond a focus on tangible things. This is a basic and key element of thought in higher education. In order to think in a complex way at the later stages of your degree, you will need to develop your ability to think in a conceptual way.

Cognitive psychologists, whose interest is in how people learn and develop thought, have put forward theories about when and how the ability to think conceptually and abstractly occurs. They tend to focus on the stages of child development: being able to understand concepts is one stage. The developmental theorist Piaget called it the stage of formal operations – the last of four.

When this stage is reached an individual can think abstractly, test problems in the mind and form complex ideas (Gross, 2010). Kolb was concerned with how people – including adults – learn. He argued that learning happens in a cycle and that abstract conceptualisation is an important stage in this. Learners move from concrete experiences to reflective observation, then to abstract conceptualisation before actively experimenting with the new understanding reached (Parker, 2010). We will consider Kolb's ideas in more depth in Chapter 6. For now, it is worth noting that moving between concrete and abstract ideas is an important part of the process of conceptual learning. There are a number of important concepts in midwifery that you will use in your studies and, at later stages of the course, analyse and critically evaluate. In this chapter our focus is on understanding them. First, we will identify some important concepts in midwifery, and then we will explore two important concepts by moving from the abstract to concrete examples and vice versa.

Concepts in midwifery

Activity 2.1	*Critical thinking*

Concepts in midwifery

Using the definition of a concept in the text above, list six concepts that you think are important in midwifery.

Below are some examples of what you might have written down.

- Normalcy.
- Choice.
- Partnership.
- Consent.
- Non-maleficence.
- Compassion.
- Autonomy.
- Trust.

In the disciplines that inform midwifery thinking – such as biology, medicine, sociology, social policy, psychology and law – there are other concepts that you might have mentioned. These are relevant to understanding midwifery so you need to be able to discuss them in an abstract and general way, as well as being able to name specific instances.

Here are examples.

- Biology: well-being, process, change.
- Medicine: intervention, risk, cause and effect, synergy, associative change, health.
- Sociology: social class, institutionalisation, inequality.
- Psychology: loss, attachment, risk, prejudice.

- Law: rights, duty, accountability.
- Social policy: welfare, modernisation, community.

When reviewing your list, check to see that all your terms, like those above, are *abstract* notions or ideas.

In order to better understand concepts we will explore two in more detail – social exclusion and partnership. We will look at each in a different way. When exploring social exclusion we will move from the abstract to the concrete, and when considering partnership we will start with the concrete and work towards the abstract.

Activity 2.2   *Critical thinking and research*

The concept of social exclusion

- First, define social exclusion.
- Next, list the attributes or characteristics of social exclusion.
- Finally, provide some concrete examples.

These are some books you could refer to.

Gordon, D, Levitas, R and Pantazis, C (2006) *Poverty and social exclusion in Britain: the millenium survey.* Bristol: The Policy Press.

Hunt, S (2004) *Poverty, pregnancy and the healthcare professional.* Edinburgh: Books for Midwives.

Kingdon, C (2008) *Sociology for midwives.* London: Quay Books.

Marmot, M (2010) *Fair society healthy lives.* London: UCL Institute of Health Equity. Available at: www.instituteofhealthequity.org/projects/fair-society-healthy-lives-the-marmot-review. (You could search specifically for maternity-related aspects of health.)

Pierson, J (2002) *Tackling social exclusion.* London: Routledge.

Sheaff, M (2005*) Sociology and health care: an introduction for nurses, midwives and allied health professionals.* Maidenhead: Open University Press.

Compare your answers with the outline below.

First, we need a *definition* of social exclusion. Pierson (2002, p7) defines social exclusion as:

> *a process that deprives individuals and families, groups and neighbourhoods of the resources required for participation in the social, economic and political activity of society as a whole.*

Identifying the attributes or characteristics of a concept can help you to develop a better understanding of it. These are the *attributes* of social exclusion.

- It is a process – the way things work in society.
- It occurs because of the impact of structural factors.

- A variety of factors can lead to social exclusion, but poverty and low income are significant.
- It happens to a minority of people in society.
- People who experience social exclusion have different life experiences and opportunities from other people, including poorer health outcomes.

Finally, we can better appreciate social exclusion by listing some concrete *examples* of groups who are socially excluded.

- Women with disabilities whose communication needs are not met in pregnancy.
- Pregnant asylum seekers who are do not understand UK maternity care and are unable to access benefits.
- Children from families on low wages whose parents cannot afford to give them money for activities with other children or mobile phones and computers to communicate with them.
- Young women who feel they won't 'fit' into antenatal education classes because they do not have a partner or they will be perceived as stupid and irresponsible.
- Older people feeling isolated in neighbourhoods that are changing rapidly.

In the above example we started from the concept of social exclusion, using abstract thinking, and moved towards concrete examples. Another way of learning to grasp concepts is to begin with concrete examples and work towards a definition.

Activity 2.3   *Critical thinking and research*

The concept of partnership

- First, think about and write down some *concrete examples* of how midwives demonstrate partnership.
- Next, list the *attributes* of partnership.
- Finally, provide a *definition* of partnership.

Below are some useful books you could refer to.

Foster, I R and Lasser, J (2010) *Professional ethics in midwifery practice*. Burlington MA: Jones and Bartlett.

Kingdon, C (2008) *Sociology for midwives*. London: Quay Books.

Raynor, M, Marshall, J and Sullivan, A (2005) *Decision making in midwifery practice*. Oxford: Churchill Livingstone.

Now compare your answers to those below.

These are some *examples* of how midwives can demonstrate partnership.

- They can listen carefully to women's experiences in order to appreciate their situation.
- They can plan births together with women.
- They can give clear and accessible information to women about possible risks and benefits.
- They can support women to negotiate with other members of the health team.

- They can find out what may be behind women's anxiety about being in hospital.
- They can share their specialist knowledge of health services.
- They can actively involve women's partners or key supporters.

The main *attributes* of partnership are that it:

- respects women as individuals;
- involves active listening;
- requires real engagement with women;
- values women's individuality;
- empathetically appreciates women's priorities;
- requires real engagement with women;
- acknowledges inequalities in women's circumstances.

This helps us to *define* the concept of partnership as working alongside and together with women to ensure individualised care.

The principles and values of midwifery

Having explored concepts, and some ways of grasping them, we will consider the principles of midwifery. The *Concise Oxford English Dictionary*, (11th edition) (2008) defines a principle as *a fundamental truth or proposition serving as the foundation for action*. So we can see that principles, like concepts, will require abstract thinking and that this can be the basis for activity. A consideration of principles also requires us to think about the nature of the profession of midwifery as distinct from others. The definition of midwifery adopted by the International Confederation of Midwives (ICM) in 2005 (and also by the World Health Organization [WHO] and the International Federation of Gynecology and Obstetrics [FIGO]) is reproduced in full in *Midwives rules and standards* produced by the Nursing and Midwifery Council (NMC, 2012) and focuses on practice spheres and practical considerations. The Royal College of Midwives' *Women centred care: position statement* (RCM, 2008a) gives more attention to principles, stating:

> *midwives encourage self-efficacy by providing a range of unbiased opinion which takes account of women's beliefs and values. This includes a non-judgemental approach to understanding that some choices or decisions made by women may not fit into our framework of institutional guidance and protocols. Nevertheless, the midwife's role remains that of being the woman's advocate by enabling her to make decisions of her own.*
> (p102)

So we can see that the RCM places importance on the principles of a non-judgemental approach: choice and autonomy are basic to midwifery.

Midwifery students are obliged to uphold the NMC (2008) *The code: standards of conduct, performance and ethics for nurses and midwives,* which sets out the conduct expected of midwives (and student midwives) – behaviour that is consistent with a set of values. Hence throughout your course you will be expected to demonstrate these values both in your assignments and in your midwifery practice during your placement. The conduct expected of students is further outlined in the NMC's *Guidance on professional conduct for nursing and midwifery students* (NMC, 2013b).

The values of midwifery

Find your copy of the NMC (2008) *The code: standards of conduct, performance and ethics for nurses and midwives* (www.nmc-uk.org). This sets out the behaviour that is expected of midwives (and nurses). From the code, put together a list of the values of midwifery expressed in an abstract way.

You might have written:

- respect for people and their dignity;
- honesty and integrity;
- confidentiality;
- rights;
- safeguarding;
- cooperation;
- non-discrimination;
- integrity;
- professionalism;
- equality;
- diversity.

Women who use maternity services and values

In 2009 The National Perinatal Epidemiology Unit surveyed more than 5,000 women to find out their views about the maternity care they received. The report is called *Delivered with care: a national survey of women's experience of maternity care* (NPEU, 2010) and can be found at:

www.npeu.ox.ac.uk/files/downloads/reports/Maternity-Survey-Report-2010.pdf

- Access this survey and draw out from it the values that women who used maternity services consider to be important. Again, list them as concepts.
- Compare this list with the one from Activity 2.4.

In your second list you might have written:

- support;
- safety;
- comfort;
- trust;

- kindness;
- respect;
- choice;
- promoting independence/self-reliance.

The two lists you have compared are similar, but, as you will have noticed, have different emphases.

Values and your studies

Values will be a consistent theme during your midwifery education. They should be integrated into all aspects of your study and thinking. You will need to show that you understand and have incorporated the values of midwifery into essays and assignments, and into your practice when you are on placement. Values will provide you with a way of thinking and criteria for evaluating the theories you are studying, the midwifery practice you are observing, the social policies you are discussing and the research studies you are exploring. (You will find more on evaluation in Chapter 4.)

Case study: using values in an essay

Nazneen chose to focus her assignment on women-centred care because she wanted to draw on her previous experience as a support worker. She read Supporting women in labour: midwifery practice guidelines *(RCM, 2008b) and noted that women have said that the four aspects of support they want in labour are emotional support, informational support, physical support and advocacy. At the start of her practice, however, she had observed one situation where the midwife was too rushed to be able to provide the level of emotional support a woman had wanted, and another where a medical professional provided information in such a way that it was confusing to the woman rather than supportive. Nazneen thought carefully about the difference between the rhetoric of values – what the Trust's policies said – and the day-to-day reality she had observed on practice placement.*

In addition, the values of midwifery should guide the language you use in your written work – both at college and on your placement – and, of course, the language you use with people who use services and with colleagues. Your choice of words should be consistent with the values of respect, dignity, empowerment, anti-discrimination, inclusion and social justice. Thompson (2006) explains the important role of language in both constructing and maintaining oppression and discrimination.

Research summary: midwives' language

Stapleton et al. (2002), through their research observations of midwives and women during antenatal consultations, noted that the language used by midwives reflected unequal power relationships rather than mutual trust and reciprocity between women and midwives. This occurred through midwives' focus on the risks rather than the benefits of non-interventionist approaches and on downplaying the limitations of technological interventions.

Language can be used in other ways – to create relationships of partnership and responsiveness with people who use services. The words with which you choose to express yourself will convey how you understand the circumstances of the people who use maternity services, and the value you place on them, together with how you see the role and purpose of midwifery.

Activity 2.6   *Communication*

Choice of words

Think about the way language can be used when supporting women and families. Consider the way in which the words and phrases below, when used by health professionals, could convey messages about power relationships with the women who are using their services.

- Allow or let.
- Ladies, girls, patients.
- Delivery (as opposed to birth).
- High risk.
- Incompetent (cervix).
- Failure to progress (labour).
- Try (as in *Do you want to try to breastfeed?* or *Do you want to try to labour without an epidural?*).

Some difficulties with values

Students can find it difficult to thoroughly integrate values in their work. In order to do it, it is important to ensure that your reading includes discussion about values.

Case study: Linda's developing understanding

Linda's first community placement gave her the opportunity to observe her mentor-run antenatal education classes in a local children's centre. Two young mothers, Dee and Jo who she had seen in antenatal clinic appointments, had been encouraged to attend the classes. In preparation, Linda had searched for some reading about supporting younger women in pregnancy (Breheny and Stephens, 2010). Only Jo attended the first class, and she left in the tea-break despite the warmth and focused support of the community midwife. Linda observed the young woman's discomfort at sitting between some very articulate and lively older couples. She had read about how young women can feel alienated by the way in which services are structured and learnt that they are sometimes actually unable to use them because of the way in which they are organised. The literature helped Linda to realise that young women had little choice about what services were available. If they did not use the services, it could be a conscious decision in order to reduce the possibility of being in a stressful situation where they might feel criticised or judged. It interested Linda that she had not appreciated this when she had worked with younger clients previously. She and her mentor made a plan to rethink their approach to younger women and provide them with more targeted support.

Linda was able to think more deeply about values. Sometimes students take a surface approach to values rather than the in-depth approach that studying midwifery requires, as discussed in Chapter 1. Here are some examples from student assignments we have read.

- It is very important that midwives show respect to the people they are working with.
- When on my placement I worked in a women-centred way.
- I have found values very useful when thinking about midwifery practice.

We can see that these statements do not tell us very much about the students' understanding. The writers have fallen into the trap of making points rather then developing arguments; they have superficially used the relevant language rather than delving deeper and thinking about meanings and relationships. In Chapter 1 we noted that these were signs of **surface learning**. Unless these statements are followed by thoughtful exploration, linked to examples, they demonstrate only that the student midwife knows that it is important to mention values.

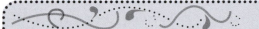

Chapter summary

This chapter has introduced the notions of concepts and principles in midwifery and provided some ways of helping you to grasp these notions. It has emphasised the importance of a sound appreciation of them as a foundation for future study and indicated the importance of a deep approach to learning. These themes will be revisited and developed in later chapters when we think further about the use of values in reflection and in evaluating research, and some of the dilemmas of implementing values in midwifery practice.

Further reading

These are useful textbooks that generally discuss midwifery and values.

Foster, I R and Lasser, J (2010) *Professional ethics in midwifery practice.* Burlington MA: Jones and Bartlett.

Kingdon, C (2008) *Sociology for midwives.* London: Quay Books.

Raynor, M, Marshall, J and Sullivan, A (2005) *Decision making in midwifery practice.* Oxford: Churchill Livingstone.

Chapter 3
Relating theory to practice

This chapter will help you to meet the Quality Assurance Agency for Higher Education (QAA, 2008) requirement that students studying at Level 4 are able to:

- demonstrate knowledge of the underlying concepts and principles associated with their area(s) of study and an ability to evaluate and interpret these within the context of that area of study;
- demonstrate an ability to present, evaluate and interpret qualitative and quantitative data in order to develop lines of argument and make sound judgements in accordance with basic theories and concepts of their subject(s) of study.

NMC Standards for Pre-registration Midwifery Education

This chapter will address the following competencies:

Domain: Achieving quality care through evaluation and research
Apply relevant knowledge to the midwife's own practice in structured ways which are capable of evaluation.

Chapter aims

After reading this chapter you will be able to:

- understand what theory is;
- appreciate the important role of theory in midwifery practice;
- identify some theories that are significant and relevant in midwifery;
- make connections between some relevant theories and midwifery thinking and practice.

Introduction

Students are required to know the underlying concepts and principles associated with their area(s) of study and interpret them within the context of that area of study. For midwifery students this means, first, being able to understand relevant and significant theories and, second, being able to explain their meaning and connections to midwifery thinking and practice. The latter is often described as linking or applying **theory** to practice – that is, showing how a theory helps to explain different aspects of midwifery. Students do not always find it easy to make these links. The purpose of this chapter is to support you in developing this academic skill.

Theory and midwifery

What is theory?

It is important first to be clear what the term theory means in an academic sense. Cottrell (2011, p149) provides a useful general definition:

A theory is a set of ideas that helps to explain why something happens or happened in a particular way, and to predict likely outcomes in the future. Theories are based on evidence and reasoning, but have not yet been conclusively proved.

Bryar and Sinclair's (2011, p27) definition is similar:

providing explanations of events, actions and phenomena.

Writing specifically about midwifery theory, Bryar and Sinclair (2011, p28) make a connection with practice:

Concepts brought together in theory provide an explanation of reality which may then be tested through observation in practice or through research.

We can see, then, that a theory is a grouping of interrelated ideas that have been systematically developed to explain not just *how* things happen and are connected but also *why*. Theories are used to illuminate, or throw light on, our understanding of issues and help us to make sense of the world. They must explain the matter logically and clearly enough for the ideas involved to be discussed, criticised and challenged.

Thompson (2000) explains that there are different levels of theories.

- Grand, macro-level or global theories (sometimes known as meta-narratives), such as Marxism or psychoanalysis, which claim to be able to explain everything in society, or all human behaviour.
- Middle-range theories, which focus on a specific set of issues rather than being able to account for things at a societal level; for instance, theories about social roles.
- Micro theories, developed to explain very small-scale situations; for instance, the relationship between a midwife and a woman on a hospital ward.

All academic subjects have a body of theory that explains the issues with which the subject is concerned. Within this there will be a range of competing theories that have different explanations for an issue. Theories can also be contested – there is not necessarily agreement about the merit of different theories. Midwifery has its own body of theory but has always drawn on other academic subjects, in particular:

- medicine: the study of health, illness and the impact of interventions;
- psychology: the study of mind and behaviour;
- sociology: the study of the relationship between the individual and their social world;
- social policy: the study of the development, implementation and impact of government health and welfare policy;
- **ethics**: the study of concepts of right and wrong and morality in relation to behaviour;
- law: the study of the relevant legislative framework and its underpinning principles.

Theories for midwives and midwifery

Midwives might use theory to understand and explain:

- the physiology and psychology of maternity and childbirth;
- ways of going about midwifery most effectively;
- the organisations within which they work;
- the lives of the women they are working with, including their internal (psychological) world and their external (social) world.

Activity 3.1   *Critical thinking*

Thinking about midwifery practice and theory

The Essential Skills Clusters for pre-registration midwifery education (NMC, 2008) set out what qualifying midwives must understand and be able to do. Read through them and draw out six specific issues in midwifery that theories might help to explain.

Below are some issues we identified. Check your list against them.

- Roles and responsibilities.
- Fetal well-being.
- Stages of pregnancy.
- Cultural and social factors.
- Exploitation, discrimination and harassment.
- Prejudices, **values** and beliefs.
- The physiology of labour and birth.
- Fear and anxiety.
- Communication.
- Bereavement.

How might theory be of use?

Midwifery, like all professions, uses theory to guide practice. Howe (2007) identifies five ways in which this might happen.

- *Observation*: theory provides guidance on what a midwife might need to look out for when working with women.
- *Description*: theory provides a generally understood and shared language in which these observations can be organised and recorded.
- *Explanation*: theory can suggest how different observations might be linked in a framework that explains them.
- *Prediction*: theory can indicate what might happen in the future.
- *Intervention*: theory can provide ideas about what might bring about a change in the situation.

Activity 3.2   *Critical thinking*

Using theory in midwifery

Paul felt privileged that his first experience of witnessing a birth as a student was at a home birth supporting Anna and her partner Yuri. As part of his preparations for the first practice module he had carried out a search on coping with pain in labour.

What theories do you think Paul might have identified?

Paul's findings

Paul found that biomedical theories of labour associated pain with suffering and dependence, and that the absence of pain appeared to be a desirable outcome. However, in the midwifery literature he found that the absence of pain was not necessarily the most important thing for women, and that satisfaction with their overall experience of labour was often a priority for them (Jones et al., 2012).

During the home birth, Paul observed how Anna had used movement and upright positions to aid progress and to feel more in control. He saw how his mentor's gentle support at critical times enhanced the efforts of the woman and her partner to be independent. This connected with his reading about the 'working with pain paradigm' where pain is accepted as an important part of the physiology of normal labour. Women use their own strategies and solutions to cope with pain, supported by appropriate, individualised care (Leap and Anderson, 2008).

Paul had also come across 'comfort' theory and was surprised to see the vast amount of literature on this aspect of care. Originating in nursing, this theory was developed to explain the complex, multidimensional needs of 'patients' in seeking comfort and the carer's role in providing or enhancing it (Kolcaba, 1994). In midwifery the strengthening role of comfort has been explored by writers who concluded that the management of pain and comfort were not necessarily synonymous (Schuiling et al., 2011).

From his reading and observations Paul concluded that theories of coping with pain in labour seemed to be inextricably linked with theories about the role of the midwife and the nature of childbirth itself. Different people reading about coping with pain might have chosen other theories. It can be useful to think about this and reflect on our preferences for some theories over others and the reasons for this.

In this chapter we will focus particularly on theories that help to explain midwifery in its current context. Many have been drawn from other disciplines, as discussed earlier. Each of these other major disciplines is made up of different 'schools', or ways of thinking about that subject, which provide contrasting ways of understanding a particular issue. For example, psychology, which offers possible explanations for human behaviour and development, is made up of different schools of thought – behaviourism, humanism, psychodynamic theory, cognitive theory and neurobiological theory (Gross, 2010). Sociology, which deals with the relationship between an individual and their social context, includes the functionalist, Marxist, interpretive, feminist and post-modernist schools (Kingdon, 2008).

It will be apparent that midwifery adopts an eclectic approach to theory. It uses theories from different disciplines so a midwife might draw on a diverse range of theories to explain a situation. Bryar and Sinclair (2011) argue that this is inevitable because there is no one global theory that can explain the complexity of the situations midwives will come across. Sometimes the term eclecticism is used unhelpfully by students and practitioners as a smokescreen for not being clear about the theoretical basis for their thinking. However, skilled and confident students and practitioners should be able to articulate their thinking and practice, drawing on a range of diverse theories in a fluent way.

In addition to the formal or official theories, discussed above, midwifery practice draws on informal 'practice' theory. Formal theories are those that can be found in academic textbooks and will be taught to you on your midwifery programme. Examples are sociological theories of health and illness, feminist theories of the division of labour in families, and biological theories of depression. Because formal theory is set out in academic books, articles and **research** studies, it can be argued about, debated, explored, analysed, tested, challenged, built on and extended. In contrast, practice theories are the ideas that midwives have developed from existing theories through their work. They are passed on from experienced staff to new recruits through day-to-day tasks and the culture of the profession. This practice wisdom that has been developed through experience and **reflection** plays an important role in developing theories for practice in midwifery. Formal theory can and should influence practice, but midwifery thinking also advances through this development of informal theories and reflection on practice (Bryar and Sinclair, 2011). This, together with Schön's (1983) notion of the reflective practitioner, will be discussed in more depth in Chapter 7.

The importance of theory

Theory is important in midwifery and midwifery education for a number of reasons.

- It is the mark of a skilled practitioner.
- It can promote accountability.

- It can help avoid discrimination.
- It provides a way of making sense of complexity and uncertainty.

The practice of all professions is based on theoretical knowledge that those working in that occupation understand, can relate to the concerns of their area of work, and are able to use to explain why they take a particular approach. Professionals need to have a shared framework for making sense of what they are observing and experiencing, and for articulating their practice. In midwifery this is essential to ensure that practice is based not on individuals' thoughts and views but on a common understanding that can be discussed and debated with colleagues.

Theory, then, provides us as midwives with a means of organising our observations and thinking, and with a shared basis on which to decide what we should be doing, what is the best way forward and why we have decided this. This means that midwives can articulate and explore with others the principles and thinking on which their practice is based and the reasons for choosing a particular approach. Explaining the theory that has guided practice in a particular direction ensures that underlying and possibly hidden assumptions can be uncovered and made clear, and, as a consequence, the reasons (the *why*) for a particular course of action can be justified. This, in turn, provides a level of accountability to colleagues, other professionals and employers. Further, being explicit and clear about the theoretical basis of your thinking and decision making also provides accountability to the people who use maternity services. It is an important element of learning to work in partnership with them.

As Bryar and Sinclair (2011, p6) argue:

> If . . . theories can be identified and discussed, they form a way of aiding communication between midwives, the childbearing woman and her family and other practitioners.

Another argument for the importance of theory is that as midwifery practice becomes increasingly complex and takes place in unpredictable and uncertain circumstances, theory provides a way of ensuring that there is a way of making sense of the multitude of experiences midwives go through each day. Midwives can become caught up in the activity of getting on with the job and forget the importance of thinking about the theoretical basis of their actions (Bryar and Sinclair, 2011). However, during your midwifery training, both in university and when on placement, it is really important to take the opportunity to take a step back from the hectic world of everyday practice, to learn and understand the theories of midwifery and to develop your ability to think theoretically.

Theory or procedures?

Some argue that there is a growing tendency for midwifery practice to be dominated by the *proliferation of policies, protocols and clinical guidelines* (Kirkham, 2010, p4). However, for a number of reasons this does not mean that theory is irrelevant (Taylor and White, 2000). First, policies and procedures are based on particular theoretical understandings. For example, if we consider the format of the antenatal booking forms that are used to assess a woman's need for social support, we see that they are linked to the *Common assessment framework* (DCSF, 2010), which is allied to the *Framework for assessment of children in need and their families* (DH, 2000), now updated by *Working together to safeguard children* (DfE, 2013). Both are derived from particular theoretical understandings of what children need from their parents to thrive and develop. The research on which this was based was set out in a related publication and made available in *The child's world* (Horwath, 2002).

Second, theory can help us to understand *why* there has been a growth in bureaucratic procedures in midwifery (and other public services). For example, Alcock (2003), writing about welfare services, notes Weber's sociological theory that explains how the internal logic of bureaucracy can become more important than the expectations of those who need to use the service. This can occur because people whose work is to ensure that procedures are followed have a vested interest in maintaining the structures and systems that are part of the bureaucracy.

Others have developed a theory of organisations called 'new managerialism' to understand the way in which the organisation of public services, including health services, changed in the late 1980s and 1990s (Alcock et al., 2008; Clarke and Newman, 1997). A significant feature of this was a focus on outputs and performance, together with attention to effectiveness. This was apparent in target setting, performance indicators to measure the achievement of targets, and the strengthening of line management. Being able to theorise organisational change can help us to appreciate the context within which the daily work of midwives takes place.

Can practice be theory-free?

In our experience, midwifery students who have been on practice placements sometimes return to university and complain that the midwives did not identify the theories they were using. Bryar and Sinclair (2011, p6) note that much *of this underlying theory . . . is hidden from discussion and view, sometimes even hidden from the person who holds them.* They have also suggested that there is strand of anti-intellectualism in midwifery that rejects the importance of theory, seeing the development of practical skills, empathy and intuition as more important (Bryar and Sinclair, 2011). However, as discussed above, behind all thoughts and behaviour are theoretical assumptions that may be hidden but are nevertheless present. This is why you will find on your course that you are asked to be clear about the theories on which you are basing your thinking and practice.

Relating theory to practice

Earlier in the chapter we noted the requirement for midwifery students to relate theory to practice. Each midwifery programme will have a different form of assessment. However, whatever form they take, you will be tested on your ability to understand principles and concepts (the theories) and interpret these within the context of midwifery. This might be through an essay, a case study, an assignment or another written piece for your portfolio of practice learning. You will be expected to show that you understand the links between theory and practice by either:

* explaining a theory and then showing how it might relate to an issue in midwifery practice; or
* considering a case study or situation you have come across in midwifery and showing how theories might help to understand it.

In the next part of the chapter, relating theory to practice in both these ways will be explored, and examples will be provided.

Theory and its relevance to midwifery practice

Before you can make that connection between a theory and practice it is important first to have a clear grasp of the theory. Without this basic understanding it will be difficult to develop your learning. It is like finding a route on a journey: if you do not understand the map, you will not be able to use to it to help you find your way. You can makes guesses about the direction you are going in, and sometimes you will be right. However, this will be accidental, and you may find yourself lost again. When you need to use this route another time, you will almost certainly find it difficult. In the same way, if you do not have a clear grasp of a theory, you will not be able to use it helpfully to make sense of what you come across in midwifery, and at later stages of the course, you will find it difficult to be critically analytic of the theory. It is worth investing the time and effort to really grasp new ideas and theories.

When applying theory to practice, it may be helpful to go about it in a step-by-step way. The stages set out below may assist you with this.

Stage one: ensure you have understood the theory

To help you understand and consider a new theory, it can be helpful to answer the following questions.

- What is this theory trying to explain?
- What discipline does it come from? How has this theory developed?
- What are the basic arguments or main points of the theory?
- Put very simply, how does the theory explain the issue?

If you do not understand the textbook you are using, it can be helpful to go back to a more basic explanation in a different book. However, you should not rely on simpler textbooks; rather, use them as steps towards understanding books or articles written at the appropriate level for your qualification. Always return to an academic source written at a level appropriate to your stage of study.

Stage two: outline the theory in your own words

Next, try to explain the theory in your own words. Aim not to use the phrases and words in the books from which you have drawn. It will be a good test of your understanding if you can write it in an original way. If you are stuck, it can be helpful to speak it out loud and write down what you have said. It also can be helpful to try to explain it to another student or even a friend – maybe someone who has little experience of midwifery. Often teaching something to someone else is a test of whether you have grasped it (Race, 2010).

Case study: Linda learns to understand theory

Linda found that though Maggie, her 'critical friend', was really helpful for checking out some issues, they tended to get each other into a muddle when they tried working together to understand theories. So Linda asked her husband Gary if it would be alright if she tried to get her thoughts together by explaining a theory, in her own words, to him. He was fine with this, and it gave Linda a great opportunity to get feedback on whether she had understood clearly. An unintended, but helpful, consequence was that Gary felt more involved in Linda's studies – whereas before he had been feeling a bit pushed out by her intense focus on the course.

Stage three: make a connection between theory and practice

Once you have grasped the theory, try to think about situations from your own life or from midwifery experience that this theory might help to explain.

Activity 3.3   *Critical thinking*

Understanding theory – attachment theory

Attachment theory, which belongs in the psychoanalytic school of psychology, is used extensively in midwifery to think about the experience of the newborn child. Use the questions and stages above to ensure that you have grasped the theory and can apply it before drawing on the answers below.

You might find the following books a helpful introduction.

*   Howe, D (2001) Attachment. In Horwath, J (ed.) *The child's world: assessing children in need.* London: Jessica Kingsley, pp194–206.
*   Kirkham, M (2010) *The midwife-mother relationship* (2nd edition). Basingstoke: Palgrave Macmillan, pp236–37.
*   Paradice, R (2002) *Psychology for midwives.* London: Quay Books, Chapters 8 and 10.
*   Raynor, M and England, C (2010) *Psychology for midwives.* Maidenhead: Open University Press, Chapter 9.
*   Redshaw, M (2006) First relationships and the growth of love. In Page, L A and McCandlish, R (eds) *The new midwifery* (2nd edition). Edinburgh: Churchill Livingstone. Chapter 2.

A possible answer to Activity 3.3

Q. What is this theory trying to explain?

A. Attachment theory aims to explain how and why children develop relationships with their caregivers and the impact on children's psychological and emotional development if they do not experience satisfactory relationships.

Q. What discipline and school of thinking does it come from? How has this theory developed?

A. Attachment theory is a theory from the psychoanalytic school of psychology. It assumes that people's behaviour is the result of interaction between motivation/drives and their environment. Current theory on attachment has evolved from John Bowlby's theories on how children respond when they are separated from their mother. These were developed by Mary Ainsworth, who observed young children with their attachment figures to see how they behaved during separation from the caregiver and when the caregiver returned. From this she devised a classification of types of attachment.

Q. What are the basic arguments or main points of the theory?

A. The theory argues that secure attachment of babies to responsive adults is an important foundation for social competence during childhood and in teenage and adult life, so relationships in very early childhood are significant for later life. Children need consistent warmth, security, responsiveness and positive, trusted attachment relationships in order to develop feelings of confidence, self-worth, emotional stability and security. Children with a negative experience of attachment figures who are unresponsive, inconsistent, unhelpful or hostile can lack self-confidence and trust, and feel insecure and anxious.

Q. Put very simply, how does the theory explain the issue?

A. People are born with a basic drive towards seeking security and protection from harm through closeness to someone who is seen as stronger and wiser – an attachment figure. While this is true for people of all ages, in later life attachments are usually more reciprocal or mutual. For young children the way caregivers respond to them comes to be their internal working model, and from this they develop a sense of how they generally expect people to respond to them. The types of parent–infant relationship most likely to be helpful to children developing secure attachment are those in which the parent responds consistently, sensitively and appropriately to the child's signals. This will include bodily closeness and giving comfort when the baby is distressed.

This possible answer refers to theorists John Bowlby and Mary Ainsworth. If you wanted to read more about their theories, you could look at:

- Bowlby. J (2003) *A secure base*. London: Routledge.
- Gross, R (2010) *Psychology: the science of mind and behaviour*. London: Hodder Education, Chapter 32.

Connecting theory and practice

> ### Case study: Nazneen connects theory to practice
>
> *Nazneen listened carefully during the session on attachment at university. At the time she was not really certain about the relevance of it, though she did reflect on how, when she was a maternity support worker, different mothers and fathers had responded to their babies in different ways. Her group was given the following question:*
>
> *What situations from midwifery might attachment theory help us to understand?*
>
> *The group worked together on this and came up with the following answers, and this really helped Nazneen to see how midwifery practice during and after birth, and within the confines of a hospital setting, draws on the insights of attachment theory.*
>
> - *The physical environment can be organised so it is easier and feels more natural for mothers to be physically close to their newborn babies.*
> - *It is seen as important that care around the time of birth is planned to minimise the separation of mothers from their babies and to promote opportunities for holding babies.*
> - *Fathers are encouraged to be involved in the birth of their babies so that they have the opportunity to be responsive parents right from the beginning of their baby's life.*
>
> *Nazneen also thought back to her experience of volunteering in a family centre with parents and their children under the age of five. She particularly remembered Delia, the mother of two-year-old Janey, who had shared her experience of childbirth in a parents' group facilitated by a family centre worker. Delia explained that after Janey was born she felt low and tired, and it was really difficult to pick her up when she cried. Fortunately, Delia had a supportive sister with whom she was able to talk. She encouraged Delia to get help with how she was feeling and spoke to Delia's partner. He was able to help – and whenever possible joined in Janey's care in a sensitive and responsive way. Nazneen was able to make a connection between her learning about attachment, Janey's experience when she was a newborn baby, what might have got in the way of her developing secure attachments, and how the family worked together to ensure her needs were met.*

Obviously, this is the 'bare bones' of attachment theory and its implications for midwifery practice. On your programme you will be expected to use a number of sources and explore the arguments of the theory in more depth. The purpose here is not to provide an extensive debate concerning attachment theory but to show how you first need to be able to grasp theory before you start to make the connections to midwifery.

Using theories to help to understand situations in midwifery

Now we will explore how you can use theories to make sense of a situation in midwifery. In order to be able to identify theories that might help you to understand a midwifery situation or case study, you need to have a 'toolkit' of theories on which you can draw. This means, as discussed above, having a good basic grasp of a range of theories.

In order to be able to think theoretically about a situation, it will be helpful to develop a disposition as an active, enquiring learner developing a deep approach to their studies. By this, we mean someone who is:

- motivated to explore an issue;
- open to learning;
- prepared to look beneath the surface and ask questions;
- curious about whatever they encounter;
- keen to understand more;
- able to think deeply;
- willing to have their ideas challenged.

Your lecturers and mentors will encourage you to develop good habits of active learning – for example, by making suggestions about exploratory questions to ask when you come across new situations. However, this cannot substitute for taking responsibility for your own personal development as a learner.

Here are some examples of questions you can ask when you are presented with a new situation in midwifery or a case study.

- What is it important to understand here because of how I feel about the situation? (Your feelings can be a guide to what is important, and it will be crucial not to discount them, but to give them careful attention.)
- What is it important to understand here in order to improve the situation?
- What theories might help me understand what is going on and from which disciplines?
- Do I need theories from psychology – which could help explain behaviour?
- Do I need theories from medicine – which could help with issues about health, illness and the impact of interventions?
- Do I need theories from sociology – which could help explain the relationship between the individual and their social context?
- Is there social policy theory that might help to explain aspects of this situation?
- How well do the theories I have identified help to explain what is going on here? How has it helped my understanding to have used theory to explain these issues?

Activity 3.4   *Critical thinking*

Linking theory to practice

Use the questions set out above to try to link theory to practice in this case study before reading the suggested answers below.

Paul and his mentor Ann visit Bryony on day six following the birth of her baby by emergency caesarean section. She seems very angry and talks at length about her experiences, saying she now feels guilty about her decision to have an epidural in labour, which she links to the need for a caesarean. She had wanted to have a water birth but says she felt pressurised into having an epidural when her blood pressure rose in early labour.

A possible answer to Activity 3.4

Q. What is it important to understand here because of how I feel about the situation?

A. You might feel upset or disconcerted by Bryony's apparent anger; you might be concerned about practical considerations, as well as the possibility of her risk of depression.

Q. What is it important to understand here in order to improve the situation?

A. It is important to understand why Bryony feels the way she does: what are her main concerns and what can be done about them? What else could be contributing to her response to her experiences?

Q. Do I need theories from psychology – which could help explain behaviour? Do I need theories from sociology – which could help explain the relationship between the individual and their social context? What theories do I need to know from obstetrics and midwifery literature to understand the mechanisms of labour and how pathology in health can interfere with process and progress?

A. From *psychology*, the 'stages of loss' theory might help to understand Bryony's anger. Briefly put, this theory argues that people who have experienced any kind of loss move through four stages before coming to terms with their loss. The stages are said to be shock, denial, anger and depression (Paradice, 2002).

From *sociology*, theories about birth technologies and the body together with feminist theory about control and body image might help to explain why Bryony was upset about not having achieved the 'perfect' birth (Kingdon, 2008; Oakley, 2005).

From *obstetric medicine* Paul can start to appreciate the issues surrounding raised blood pressure in labour and how midwives respond to changes in health status. He needs to build on his knowledge of pain relief in labour, the effectiveness of different types and their effect on the woman and baby and the progress of the labour (Jones et al., 2012). He might also think about his earlier reading on comfort and pain relief and contrast Bryony's experience of pain relief with the experience of Anna, the woman in the home birth referred to in Activity 3.2.

Q. How well do the theories I have identified help to explain what is going on here? How has it helped my understanding to have used theory to explain these issues?

A. Bryony's anger might be understood as a normal stage that she will need to go through before she adjusts to her situation, rather than as her being dissatisfied with you or the maternity services. It might suggest that she will enter a stage of depression before she is able to come to terms with the loss she has experienced. In addition, it might also help you to think about what midwifery approaches are likely to be most helpful to support her through this.

While we can see how theories can provide ways of helping to understand some aspects of Bryony's situation, it is also important to consider their limitations. Although a theory is set out in a textbook, it may still receive criticism. There are disagreements about most theories, and it is a characteristic of your developing learning that you recognise that all knowledge is contestable (Moon, 2008). For instance, the stage theory of loss – which we used above to explain Bryony's anger – has been disputed. The main points of criticism are the following.

- The theory assumes that everybody must go through all the fixed stages in order to achieve adjustment.
- Many people's experiences are not accounted for by the theory; in particular, no consideration is given to differences arising from gender or ethnicity.
- Loss is more complex than the theory allows for.
- There are competing theories that suggest that after loss the way people reconstruct meaning depends on contextual factors – not pre-set stages.
  (Oliver and Sapey, 2006; Paradice, 2002)

A major criticism of traditional theories from the social sciences is that they have been developed from a white male, able-bodied, middle-class, heterosexual and eurocentric perspective – and hence may not adequately explain issues in a diverse and stratified society made up of both men and women (Abbott et al., 2005; Robinson, 2008; Williams, 1989). Furthermore, theories cannot determine or dictate what a midwife's approach to practice might be – each situation is unique, and the individuality of a woman should be an essential factor in planning how to proceed. Theory must be coupled with values, reflection, **analysis** and a critical stance. In your studies at higher levels of the degree you will be required to take a more analytic, critical and reflective approach to theories, and this will be explored in later chapters, particularly Chapters 5 and 11.

Chapter summary

This chapter has highlighted the requirement that midwifery students during the first level of the degree should be able to apply relevant theories to the concerns and practice of midwifery. To assist you in this, the chapter has clarified what theory is, how everything has theoretical foundations, and the important role played by theory. Frameworks for applying theory to practice and understanding practice situations theoretically have been suggested and some examples provided.

Despite its importance, you will be aware that using theory is not the only component of effective practice. Other essential ingredients are: knowledge of procedures and legislation; the integration of values; learning from the knowledge and experience of people who use services; working in a skilled manner; using research to inform practice; and building practice wisdom through reflection. However, being able to relate theory to practice as discussed in this chapter will provide you with an important foundation that can enhance your understanding of the other aspects of practice and on which you will need to build at a later stage in your studies. In Parts Two and Three these issues will be developed further.

Further reading

Theory

Bryar, R and Sinclair, M (eds) (2011) *Theory for midwifery practice* (2nd edition). Basingstoke: Palgrave Macmillan.

A thorough and helpful exploration of the use of theory in midwifery practice.

Thompson, N (2000) *Theory and practice in human services* (2nd edition). Maidenhead: Open University Press.

This book is useful for a more in-depth discussion of the relationship between theory and practice, although, as the title suggests, it covers the human services generally – not only midwifery.

Pain management

Jones L, Othman, M, Dowswell, T, Alfirevic, Z, Gates, S, Newburn, M, Jordan, S, Lavender, T and Neilson, J P (2012) *Pain management for women in labour: an overview of systematic reviews*. Cochrane Database of Systematic Reviews 2012, Issue 3. Art. no. CD009234. DOI: 10.1002/14651858.CD009234. pub2.

Kirkham, M (2010) The maternity services context. In Kirkham, M (ed.) *The midwife–mother relationship* (2nd edition). Basingstoke: Palgrave Macmillan.

Kolcaba, K (1994) A theory of holistic comfort for nursing. *Journal of Advanced Nursing*, 19 (6): 1178–84.

Leap N and Anderson, P (2008) The role of pain in normal birth and the empowerment of women. In Downe, S (ed.) *Normal childbirth: evidence and debate* (2nd edition). London: Churchill Livingstone.

Schuiling, K D, Sampselle C and Kolcaba, K (2011) Exploring the presence of comfort within the context of childbirth. In Bryar, R and Sinclair, M (eds) *Theory for midwifery practice* (2nd edition). Basingstoke: Palgrave Macmillan.

Chapter 4
Writing academically

Evaluation, developing arguments, avoiding pitfalls

This chapter will help you to meet the Quality Assurance Agency for Higher Education (2008) requirement that students studying at Level 4 are able to:

- demonstrate an ability to present, evaluate and interpret qualitative and quantitative data, in order to develop lines of argument and make sound judgements in accordance with basic theories and concepts of their subject(s) of study;
- communicate the results of their study/work accurately and reliably with structured and coherent arguments;
- evaluate the appropriateness of different approaches to solving problems related to their area(s) of study and/or work.

NMC Standards for Pre-registration Midwifery Education

This chapter will address the following competencies:

Domain: Effective midwifery practice
Complete, store and retain records of practice.

Chapter aims

After reading this chapter you will be able to:

- improve your ability to present your thinking clearly;
- appreciate how to evaluate concepts and data;
- understand how to develop structured and coherent arguments;
- know how to avoid some pitfalls in writing academically.

Introduction

This chapter is about the skills needed in written assignments at Level 4 of the degree in midwifery. Assignments will be designed in different ways depending on the programme. However, in all written forms of assessment you will be required to present ideas clearly, using language appropriate to academic study. Assignments will also test your ability to evaluate both **quantitative** data and **qualitative** concepts and to explain your thinking in structured arguments.

Aspects of writing

Some midwifery students are familiar with writing reports and case notes in their previous employment, and are articulate in classroom discussion and debate, but find it difficult to convey their ideas in writing.

Case study: Linda

Linda felt anxious about returning to writing academic assignments. She found she had lots of ideas and, in her head, knew what she might want to put into the assignments – especially issues arising from her observation of midwifery practice. These were all recorded in her reflective diary. However, when she began writing assignments, she found it difficult to use her reading and organise her thinking to convey what she wanted to say. Her tutor encouraged her to be selective and not to try to include everything in one assignment. She suggested that Linda might be more systematic about taking notes from reading and research, and think more carefully about the connection between her reading and her observations. Linda found this helpful. Learning more about structuring and organising was also useful when she was making clinical notes on the ward.

Case study: Nazneen

Nazneen's recent experience of studying at A level stood her in good stead when tackling her first assignment. She felt she was able to build on what she had learnt about organising her thoughts and selecting relevant material from her reading. It was more challenging for her to make the connections between her academic studies and the practice of midwifery. However, with guidance and a practical example from her tutor she began to see how the links could be made.

Linda and Nazneen learnt a useful lesson – that some skills, which may appear to be purely academic, can be used in other settings. These are known as transferable skills. Many skills that you will develop and use in university will be helpful to you on placement.

When thinking about writing it can be helpful to be clear about different kinds of writing and their purposes. At this level of the degree you are expected to be able to use descriptive and evaluative writing and to be able to put forward a developed argument. In the next part of the book (Chapter 5) we will explore how to write in a critical and analytic way.

Descriptive writing

Descriptive writing is needed to give important and relevant background information so that the rest of the written piece of work makes sense. It is normally best to keep this to a minimum so that you have plenty of words left for other more complex types of writing. Descriptive writing is used to:

- give information;
- list detail;
- state what something is like;
- give the order of events;
- explain what a theory says;
- set out the approach used;
- say when something occurred;
- list different aspects of a situation;
- state different options;
- explain connections between items.

In essay titles, or the instructions for assignments, the words *outline, explain, present, state* and *describe* indicate that what is expected is descriptive writing. This is often required so tutors can assess whether you are able to identify and understand the main aspects of an issue or, put another way, your grasp of propositional knowledge (as outlined in Chapter 2). A sound foundation of knowledge that makes sense to you is essential for the development of a deeper learning approach later in your degree (Biggs and Tang, 2011).

Because, when studying for a degree, you are expected to do more than describe, the instruction to 'describe' is generally followed by an instruction to write in a different way – often to evaluate or criticise.

Case study: a student assignment

Many factors influence parents' experience of childbearing and childbirth.

(a) Outline two factors you consider to be important.

(b) Evaluate the potential for the midwife to positively influence these factors.

Draw on your reading and your practice observations in your answer.

In this assignment we can see some of the uses of descriptive writing. In (a), students are asked to outline *two factors they consider to be important, drawing on both their reading and their observations. However, in (b),*

continued . . .

they are asked to think more deeply and to evaluate, or weigh up, the potential for midwives to influence these factors. First, we will think about descriptive writing by focusing on Linda's answer to part (a).

The two factors Linda chose to focus on were antenatal classes and the birth environment. She had memories of antenatal classes herself and, as part of her studies, had observed a midwife running some classes. She drew on her background reading – the list of references can be found at the end of this chapter.

Here is the beginning of Linda's answer to part (a) in which she writes about antenatal classes:

Many women are keen to attend antenatal classes when they are having their first baby and feel it is an important part of their experience of pregnancy and the maternity care provided. Antenatal classes can give them the opportunity to find out more about services they can access, including how to get support and advice in pregnancy and as new parents. One important aspect I noticed was how women used classes to reduce their anxieties about pregnancy and labour, and, in particular, birth. They were very keen to learn how to cope with a new baby. Some women also look forward to meeting other women and their families, to share experiences and give each other mutual support.

Antenatal education has moved away from an old-fashioned classroom-type approach – where standard information is given out – towards more participative sessions where the agenda is set by those attending and where there is more of an attempt to involve women and their supporters in activities that are useful and meaningful. There is, however, a great deal of public health information that the midwife is obliged to share with women, and I noticed that the midwives were skilled in conveying this while avoiding a 'tick-box' approach. In the antenatal clinics, women in early pregnancy were given information about choices for the place of birth. Some seemed surprised that home birth was offered as a choice, but the discussion of the advantages and disadvantages suggested that the home was a suitable and safe environment.

Activity 4.1 — *Reflection*

Recognising descriptive writing

Identify which parts of Linda's answer correspond to the features of descriptive writing listed above.

Activity 4.2 — *Decision making*

Descriptive writing

List, using bullet points, the main descriptive points you would include in an answer about the second factor Linda chose – the environment of childbirth. You could draw on the reading listed at the end of this chapter to assist you.

A possible answer

The environment influences parents' experience of childbirth in the following ways.

- The different environments in midwifery led units (MLUs) and a hospital setting will impact on parents' experiences. There is sound evidence that continuity of carer in labour has a positive effect on the birth outcome. The birth environment might be important in more ways than just the décor and the ambience.
- The facilities in the birthing environment can encourage the woman to be upright and mobile – for example, the provision of a pool, birthing stools, birthing couches, mats and birthing balls. These may promote the progress of labour, reduce the need for pain relief and, if an epidural is used, reduce associated problems in the second stage.
- The design and layout of the birthing environment can help the woman and her partner feel more relaxed and comfortable. This can be achieved by an environment that is as non-clinical as possible, where the bed is not prominent, calm and soothing colours and textures are used and the furniture is comfortable for the woman and her family.
- The atmosphere of the birth environment may enable the woman to labour more peacefully and encourage natural oxytocin production.
- The culture of the environment might impact on the midwife and other carers. That midwives work more independently in the MLUs can have an effect on the labouring woman, keeping her on a normal pathway. Midwives might be less likely to be pulled away to carry out additional tasks. All this can encourage independent decision making, continuity of carer and a focus on the woman and her family.

When you are using descriptive writing you will find that it is important to:

- aim to write clearly and succinctly so that you do not take up too much of an assignment with description;
- focus on the most relevant aspects of the issue you are describing – this means you will need to appreciate what is important and be able to pull out from your reading the main and most essential points;
- keep a clear focus – not drifting off the point;
- think about the most helpful order in which to present the information.

Evaluative writing

To evaluate means to *weigh up* or *assess*, to look for the *strengths* and *weaknesses*, the *positives* and the *negatives*. Other **evaluation** words you might find in assignment titles are *appraise*, *compare* and *contrast*. In your assignments you might be asked to evaluate an experience, an argument, a theory, midwifery practice, a policy, an issue or a set of statistics. This will involve making a judgement about the worth, usefulness or validity of what it is you are evaluating.

Case study: Linda's assignment

If we return to Linda's assignment, we can see that in (a) she is asked to outline. In answering (b) she has the opportunity to evaluate the potential for the midwife to positively influence the factors that impact on childbearing and childbirth.

Here is Linda's answer to (b) in which she evaluates the role of the midwife in antenatal classes:

I consider the role of the midwife to be really important in relation to antenatal classes. It begins with the way they encourage prospective parents to attend the classes – how they describe the classes and their usefulness. How they do this might persuade people who are reluctant that classes could be helpful.

If the midwife who facilitates the classes is open and welcoming, the classes are likely to be more relaxed. From observing my mentor in these sessions, I know it can be a challenge to meet the needs of a diverse, sometimes quite large, group of people. Among the groups of parents-to-be I could see there were varying levels of knowledge and experience on all aspects of pregnancy, childbirth and parenting, so it was demanding to engage them in discussions and encourage them all to participate in activities.

The midwife can affect how much parents learn from the class. My mentor had found that parents were very keen to be given lots of information about future life with a baby – not just practical baby care information, but anticipating anxieties and difficult emotions. She told me that she had learnt that it was important not to leave this topic to the last class but to include elements in every session (Schott and Priest, 2002). Nolan (1998) points out that parenting does not start after the birth of the baby: the woman is already nurturing her baby, and she and her supporter may be forming a relationship by talking to and responding to their baby's movements. Parents are already making lots of decisions which will affect their baby's life, and I observed my mentor tuning into this by offering information on health promotion and emotional well-being throughout the antenatal period in clinics as well as in classes. She worked hard to involve fathers and pointed out positive male role models and behaviours in subtle ways in the videos that she used in group work. She had also, in the past, run fathers-only sessions using a male facilitator. Although this had proved popular it was curtailed by cost cutting (Symon and Lee, 2003).

Midwives can positively influence parents' experience through using their communication skills to ensure people attending feel they are valued. My mentor ran a group for younger mothers that progressed from being a forum for antenatal advice and information into a postnatal support group. She displayed impressive listening skills when interacting with this lively group, who eventually had plenty to say but initially contributed very little. I talked with the young women and asked them what they liked or did not like about the group. Their feedback on the midwife was 'great', 'she understands what its like', she doesn't judge us', 'she really listens and that helps me'. I concluded that my mentor's careful approach to communication demonstrated the potential for midwives to really make a difference to the experience of women and their families.

Criteria to use when evaluating

When evaluating, you need to use criteria or principles to help you weigh the issues. These might be:

- relevant theories;
- research evidence;
- statistics;
- midwifery values;
- your observations;
- the perspectives of women;
- personal experience.

Some of these will carry more weight than others. For example, while the use of personal experience is valued on midwifery programmes, and can convey powerfully aspects of real life, it represents the understanding of one person. In comparison, a piece of research might have involved a survey of 1,000 people and have breadth – though not depth.

Activity 4.3   *Critical thinking*

Criteria for evaluation

Identify the criteria Linda used to evaluate the potential of midwives in antenatal classes:

Comment

First Linda used her own *observations* of how prospective parents responded to the skilful way in which the midwife ran the antenatal classes and her observations of the skills used by the midwife.

She listened to what the *young women told her about their experiences* of being in the antenatal class that was also a support group.

She drew on her *reading* about parents' approaches to pregnancy and what is helpful when planning antenatal classes.

She drew on her knowledge about basic *counselling theory*, which suggests that people can be helped if they feel well listened to (Rogers, 1961).

Below is a list of questions that you could use to help you evaluate.

- What are the strengths/positives?
- Why are these positives?
- What are the limitations/weaknesses?
- Why are these limitations?
- What was not covered? What gaps are there?
- What aspects of social inclusion were considered?
- What aspects of social inclusion were not taken into account?
- Were the values of midwifery integrated?

Activity 4.4   *Critical thinking*

Evaluative thinking

In order to develop your evaluative thinking, identify three aspects of the positive potential for midwives to influence the birth environment, and then identify three limitations.

Below are some points concerning the *positive potential* you might have identified.

- Midwives can give advice about what is a helpful environment, and their guidance may be listened to and taken up by parents.
- Midwives can adapt the environment within which women are giving birth and strive to ensure that the environment does not negatively impact on the care that is offered. Even when there is a need for continuous monitoring, it is possible for women to be upright and mobile. The lighting can always be adjusted and the furniture moved to provide the most positive and nurturing environment possible.
- In a busy environment such as a delivery suite, midwives can be the guardian of the woman's privacy and dignity, limiting the level of intrusion in the room and providing continuity of care as far as possible.
- There is the potential for midwives to influence design and planning of new services.

Below are some points concerning the *limitations* you might have identified.

- Institutional constraints in a traditionally designed delivery suite may limit the midwife's ability to be creative in shaping the environment to be woman friendly. For example, the hospital may limit who can be present at the birth or dictate how the midwife and the woman's supporters occupy the space.
- Midwives may need to respond to a woman's changing health status in labour or an increase in risk factors. This may necessitate a change in environment or may limit or alter the environment. (For example, sudden blood loss in labour may entail a move from an MLU or the introduction of monitoring.)
- In home births, the midwife may be limited in her ability to influence the environment due to the physical constraints of the home.

Later in the chapter we will consider making judgements based on an evaluation.

Evaluating data

You will find that you also need to be able to evaluate data presented to you. This data will often be presented in the form of a table of statistics.

Case study: evaluating statistics

The students on Nazneen's course have been asked to select a set of statistics and to:

- *outline the information contained in the statistics;*
- *evaluate the usefulness of the statistics.*

Nazneen has decided to study some breastfeeding initiation figures to find out if rates are improving and whether there are regional variations. She compares the north-east, where she lives, to London and the overall England figures (see Table 4.1).

Period	2006/07	2007/08	2008/09	2009/10	2010/11
England	68.10%	69.90%	71.70%	72.70%	73.70%
London	79.20%	83.20%	83.80%	84.20%	86.40%
North-east	49.30%	52.40%	54.40%	55.60%	57.70%

Period	2010/11 Q1	2010/11 Q2	2010/11 Q3	2010/11 Q4	2011/12 Q1	2011/12 Q2
England	73.40%	73.70%	73.50%	73.90%	74.30%	74.10%
London	85.30%	86.3%	86.90%	86.50%	87.70%	86.90%
North-east	56.90%	56.90%	58.20%	58.50%	58.50%	57.90%

Table 4.1 Trends in initiation of breastfeeding by PCT and SHA (some regional extracts)

Source: DH (2012) and available at www.dh.gov.uk/en/Publicationsandstatistics/Publications/PublicationsStatistics/DH_130857 (Crown Copyright)

In her outline description of the figures she made the following points.

- *The figures for the years 2006–2009/10 are presented as annual figures. Since 2010/11 the figures are broken down into each quarter of the year.*
- *The overall trend is an increase in the breastfeeding initiation rate in the last five- to six-year period. The initiation rate is nearly 75 per cent for the whole of England.*
- *Regional variations are marked when the north-east is compared to London and England as a whole.*
- *A slight decrease is evident in the last quarter for the North-east and for England overall, but this pattern can be seen in previous years and does not necessarily indicate an ongoing downward trend.*

continued . . .

In Nazneen's evaluation of the statistics she made the following points about the strengths of the statistics.

- *The figures are clearly set out, and the use of percentages enables comparisons to be made.*
- *The shift to quarterly figures is helpful and might enable Trusts and care providers to more closely analyse the effectiveness of any initiatives introduced to increase rates of breastfeeding.*
- *Low rates of breastfeeding are generally linked to poverty and social disadvantage. These figures showing lower rates in the North-east of England, a relatively deprived area, support this.*

Nazneen made the following points about the weaknesses of the statistics.

- *The exact definition of breastfeeding initiation is not provided.*
- *The figures do not show for how long women continued to breastfeed.*
- *Figures are provided for two regions only. More meaningful comparisons could be made if a wider range was included.*

In order to identify the second point under strengths, Nazneen needed to be aware that considerable public health attention has been aimed at increasing rates of breastfeeding. To be able to identify the third strength, she needed an understanding of the relationship between socio-economic indicators and aspects of health. In order to identify the first two weaknesses, Nazneen would need to draw on her prior knowledge of breastfeeding, including the importance of breastfeeding and the professional language used to describe it. She would need to have asked the questions What is missing? *and* What are the gaps?

This demonstrates that background knowledge, a systematic approach to evaluation and a strong awareness of relevant issues are all needed. If you want to explore the issues behind these figures in more depth, you might find the study by Dyson et al. (2006) helpful. Details are given in the Further reading list at the end of this chapter.

Nazneen had noticed broad socio-economic differences between mothers who intended to start breastfeeding and those who were clear they wanted to bottle-feed. This was consistent with the regional socio-economic trends indicated in the statistics and led her to reflect more on the significance of socio-economic factors. She read another systematic research summary: NICE (2005) Breastfeeding for longer – what works? *A finding that interested her was that 'disadvantaged groups' were not a homogenous entity. Different groups viewed breastfeeding in different ways. For example, women from black and ethnic minority groups tended to have higher rates of breastfeeding initiation and continuation rates but might also have higher rates of early mixed feeding. Nazneen learnt that the statistics she had evaluated needed more in-depth analysis and that reading more on the topic could help her to understand the limitations of statistics.*

Developing an argument in a structured and coherent way

If you are new to academic writing, it will help you to present your evaluative thinking if you develop the skill of putting your arguments in a structured and coherent way. Below are some important aspects of this.

Build your argument in stages

- Start off by indicating what your overall conclusion is.
- Then set out the points that support your conclusion. For each of your points explain the evidence you have drawn on to support it. You will need to indicate where the evidence is drawn from and be confident that it has validity.
- Next, set out some points that provide a different point of view from your conclusion. Again, you should explain the evidence you have drawn on, its sources and its validity.
- Now that you have set out both sides of the argument and the supporting evidence, explain clearly why you have chosen one view rather than another.
- Try to ensure that the points you make follow logically from each other so that the reader can follow your argument.

It can be helpful to aim for paragraphs of roughly equal length, each containing a main theme, as this can break up the text of an assignment into manageable ideas. When you become more confident with academic writing you might vary their size, but paragraphs rarely contain fewer than two or three sentences. Aim to avoid long, confusing sentences; it can be helpful to divide them up into two shorter ones. Try not to make too many points in one sentence. Another way to avoid lengthy sentences is to think about whether you can make your point equally well using fewer words.

Use signposting and linking words

Signposting means telling the reader where you are going with your argument. Particular words can help you both to link your ideas together and to signal to the reader where your argument is going.

Below are some useful examples of words and how they can help you construct your argument.

- *Also, in addition, then, together with, moreover*: indicate you are adding to a point already made.
- *For example, in other words, for instance, namely, particularly, as follows*: can be used to introduce examples.
- *In contrast, on the other hand, in comparison, conversely, alternatively, although*: signpost that you are introducing a different argument.
- *Therefore, hence, it can be seen that, so, consequently*: are used to introduce the result of something.
- *In short, overall, to summarise, therefore, in brief*: show that you are summarising.
- *In conclusion, to conclude, thus*: are terms to introduce the conclusion.

Write clearly

It is important to develop the skill of writing using your own words and in formal but straightforward and clear language. Putting ideas in your own words will show the reader that you have understood what you have read. It is important to avoid using colloquial or informal slang that you might use in everyday conversation. You will need to use professional terminology from midwifery, but be cautious about using jargon expressions that you have not explained, and aim to avoid unnecessary shorthand. Always use language that conveys the values of midwifery and avoids bias, discrimination and oppression, as discussed in Chapter 1. To check the clarity of your writing it can be helpful to read it out loud to yourself a day or so after you have finished the draft. This can help you to pick up basic errors and ensure it makes clear sense.

Referencing

To enable the reader of your essay or assignment to check out the sources of your argument, you need to provide references within your essay or assignment. This will make it clear that you are not claiming that someone else's ideas are your own, as this is **plagiarism**, a serious academic offence (discussed later in the chapter). You also need to provide a list of the sources you have used at the end of the essay/assignment. You should follow the referencing system that your programme specifies.

It is really helpful, and will save a lot of time, if you are organised and systematic about referencing from the beginning of your studies. Whenever you are working on an assignment it is helpful to open a new document in which you list the references you have used. When you are working on your assignment and you include a reference, add it to your list straight away. If you are including a quotation from the book or article, note the page number. As you proceed through the programme, you might also find it useful to build up an overall list of references of all the sources you have used. This can be helpful when you want to return to a book or article you have read before.

Making sound judgements

After evaluating or weighing up arguments or theories you will need to make a judgement or a conclusion about the issues you have been exploring. This should include your informed opinion, which follows logically from the points you made earlier.

Activity 4.5   *Decision making*

Coming to a judgement

Return to Linda's assignment – covered in Activity 4.2 and the following case study. Look at the list of positives and limitations, and write a brief summary in which you come to a judgement about the potential of the midwife to influence the birth environment.

Below is a possible answer:

The midwife has the potential to positively influence the birth environment. Limitations on her doing this include: complications of labour; institutional constraints; poorly designed birth facilities; the choices of women and families in their own homes. However, the midwife who understands the importance of the birth environment can always work positively with the woman and family to plan the best possible care, and use her experience, skills and imagination to make the most of the circumstances and the materials available. In doing this, the midwife is practising in a way consistent with the NMC Code (NMC, 2008, p3): make the care of people your first concern, treating them as individuals and respecting their dignity.

Some pitfalls in writing academically

Plagiarism

Plagiarism is taking the work of another person or people and using it as if it were your own, not acknowledging the source of your information or inspiration. It is regarded as a form of cheating. Your programme will have its own procedures for identifying plagiarism and procedures for dealing with it. Plagiarism can include the following.

- Lifting verbatim (word for word) written material from books and articles (including internet sites) without acknowledging where you took it from. If you are going to use the author's exact words, you must indicate that this is a direct quote. It is not acceptable to use the author's words, change a few and include it in your essay or assignment as if you had written it.
- Re-writing or paraphrasing passages from books and articles without acknowledging the source. It is important always to reference the books and articles that you have used to present information or make an argument.

Case study

Paul was trying to paraphrase findings from the Birthplace in England study *to explain an aspect of safety in relation to place of birth. He included his experience of a recent home birth (involving parents Jane and Nick) into his writing. To avoid plagiarism he considered inserting the quotation in inverted commas thus:*

'Women with planned births at home or in freestanding or alongside midwifery units were significantly less likely than those with planned births in obstetric units to have an instrumental or operative delivery or to receive medical interventions such as augmentation, epidural or spinal analgesia, general anaesthesia, or episiotomy and significantly more likely to have a "normal birth"' (Brocklehurst et al., 2011, p4).

He could have written this direct quotation in another way:

The Birthplace in England Collaborative Group (Brocklehurst et al., 2011, p4) concluded that:

> Women with planned births at home or in freestanding or alongside midwifery units were significantly less likely than those with planned births in obstetric units to have an instrumental or operative delivery or to receive medical interventions such as augmentation, epidural or spinal analgesia, general anaesthesia, or episiotomy and significantly more likely to have a 'normal birth'.

However, he chose to put the ideas into his own words. This is a much better way of writing as it shows he has read and understood the argument and can reword it.

The recent Birthplace in England study *provides significant evidence for women and clinicians about the comparative safety of different places of birth (Brocklehurst et al., 2011). This large prospective cohort study found that women who planned to have their babies at home, or in midwifery-led units, had lower rates of interventions compared to women who gave birth in obstetric units. This included major outcomes such as caesareans, instrumental births and other interventions that are of concern to women – such as epidurals and episiotomies. My mentor discussed with me how important this study was for midwives supporting families with these decisions, giving them more confidence to keep women on low-risk pathways and increasing levels of normal birth.*

Other ways of avoiding plagiarism include:

- developing the habit of making notes from books in your own words, paraphrasing the ideas of the author;
- keeping a very careful note of the source of your arguments and ideas so you do not inadvertently use the author's words;
- ensuring you fully understand the referencing system used on your course;
- referencing your written work comprehensively – then you will be sure that you have indicated the sources you have used.

Students who plagiarise the work of others, rather than taking the time and effort to really understand issues for themselves, are not making the most of their opportunities to learn and develop key academic skills. They will therefore not have fully grown into the effective thinkers they need to be in the complex world of midwifery practice.

Not building on feedback from previous assignments

There is evidence that using feedback from written assignments is very significant in developing deep and effective learning (Biggs and Tang, 2011; Gibbs, 2010). The purpose of feedback is not only to comment on the work that has been assessed but also to provide guidance for future written work – to 'feed-forward' (Race, 2010, p105). However, students can tend to focus only on the mark they have received, especially if the grade awarded was low, and not read and assimilate the written comments. If they do read them, they may not understand them and often do not act on them (Burke, 2007; McCann and Saunders, 2008). While initially you may find your tutor's comments distressing – one student confessed she had thrown hers across the room in disappointment – it will be helpful to return to the feedback when you are calm, and identify what you can learn from it. Check that you understand what your tutor has written. If you do not, ask to meet with them so you can discuss it. Pick out the major themes in the feedback, and think about what steps you need to take to develop in these areas. Responding to feedback actively and constructively can assist you both in improving your work and in your confidence to do so – self-efficacy (Biggs and Tang, 2011; Race, 2010).

Silly mistakes

Always leave yourself enough time to read through and check your work before you hand it in. This space and distance can help you to see errors that you were not able to see earlier because you were too 'close' to the assignment. Some space can help objectivity. Aim to read it through in different ways: first, ask yourself if it makes sense; then look only for spelling errors; then just check for grammar and punctuation; and finally check the referencing.

When checking for sense, questions you can ask yourself include the following.

- Do my sentences convey what I want to say?
- Have I 'signposted' the essay – i.e. have I indicated to the reader where I am taking them throughout the essay?
- Are the paragraph breaks in the right place?
- Is the argument put together in a way that makes sense?

It can be useful to find a friend to help with this as they may – seeing it for the first time – be more able to look at the assignment in a clear way.

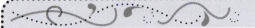

Chapter summary

This chapter has focused on some important skills in academic writing: presenting, evaluating and making judgements on concepts and data. The examples and activities provided have given you the opportunity to try out these skills in a step-by-step way. We have also considered some pitfalls in academic writing and ways of avoiding them. You will need to continue to practise and develop these skills in order to successfully progress in your studies. Without basic competence in the ability to organise your thinking and present it clearly, it will be difficult to achieve what will be required of you at the next level of the degree.

Further reading

Cottrell, S (2013) *The study skills handbook* (4th edition). Basingstoke: Palgrave Macmillan.

Dyson, L, Renfrew, M, McFadden, A, McCormick, F, Herbert, G and Thomas, J (2006) *Promotion of breastfeeding initiation and duration. Evidence into practice briefing.* London: Public Health Collaborating Centre on Maternal and Child Nutrition on behalf of the Health Development Agency (HDA) (published after the functions of the HDA were transferred to the National Institute for Health and Clinical [Care] Excellence (NICE). Available at: www.nice.org.uk/niceMedia/pdf/EAB_Breastfeeding_final_version.pdf).

Northedge, A (2005) *The good study guide* (2nd edition). Buckingham: Open University Press.

Peck, J and Coyle, M (2005) *Write it right: a handbook for students.* Basingstoke: Palgrave Macmillan.

These are useful study skills guides. Stella Cottrell's book is especially helpful and detailed. They are written for all students so they do not specifically focus on the midwifery degree.

The references for the background reading Linda used for her assignment

Brocklehurst, P et al. (Birthplace in England Collaborative Group) (2011) Perinatal and maternal outcomes by planned place of birth for healthy women with low risk pregnancies: the Birthplace in England national prospective cohort study *British Medical Journal*, 343: d7400: 1–13.

DH (Department of Health) (2011) *Preparation for birth and beyond: a resource pack for leaders of community groups and activities* London: DoH. Available at: www.dh.gov.uk/en/Publicationsandstatistics/Publications/PublicationsPolicyAndGuidance/DH_130565.

Healthcare Commission (2007) *Women's experiences of maternity care in the NHS in England: key findings from a survey of NHS trusts carried out in 2007* London: Commission for Healthcare Audit and Inspection.

NCT (2011) *Preparing for birth and parenthood: report on first-time mothers and fathers attending NCT antenatal courses.* London: NCT.

NICE (2008) *Antenatal care: routine care for the healthy pregnant woman.* London: National Institute for Health and Clinical [Care] Excellence. Available at: http://publications.nice.org.uk/antenatal-care-cg62.

Nolan, M (1998) *Antenatal education: a dynamic approach.* London: Balliere Tindall.

Royal College of Midwives (2012) *Campaign for Normal Birth: resources.* Available at: www.rcmnormalbirth.org.uk/home/.

Schott, J and Priest, J (2002) *Leading antenatal classes.* Oxford: Books for Midwives.

Part Two

Chapter 5
Developing critical analysis and understanding

This chapter will help you to meet the Quality Assurance Agency for Higher Education (QAA, 2008) requirement that students studying at Level 5 are able to:

- demonstrate knowledge and critical understanding of the well-established principles of their area(s) of study, and of the way in which those principles have developed;
- use a range of established techniques to initiate and undertake critical analysis of information, and to propose solutions to problems arising from that analysis;
- effectively communicate information, arguments and analysis in a variety of forms to specialist and non-specialist audiences, and deploy key techniques of the discipline effectively.

NMC Standards for Pre-registration Midwifery Education

This chapter will address the following competencies:

Domain: Achieving quality care through evaluation and research
Apply relevant knowledge to the midwife's own practice in structured ways which are capable of evaluation. This will include:

- critical appraisal of knowledge and research evidence;
- critical appraisal of the midwife's own practice.

Chapter aims

After reading this chapter you should be able to:

- explain what is meant by critical thinking;
- develop your critically analytic thinking and writing
- apply critical analysis to a midwifery issue.

Introduction

At this stage of the degree, undergraduate students are expected to be able to use critical thinking to understand their subject, to analyse issues and to propose solutions. In addition they should be able to communicate all this effectively. During the rest of your degree studies you will be expected to continue to develop and enhance your ability to think critically in order to explore issues of greater complexity. In this chapter we will explore what is meant by critical thinking in the academic world – the challenges it poses, the stages of development and how to develop this aptitude.

What is critical thinking?

The outline below combines and synthesises some ideas about the ingredients of critical thinking.

Concept summary: Critical thinking

Critical thinking involves the following.

- Taking a questioning and sceptical stance.
- Aiming for a deep understanding of knowledge and complex ideas. This includes an appreciation of the context of the ideas, their history, their construction, their relationship to other knowledge. This means not seeing knowledge as a series of facts.
- Exploring a range of alternative ideas.
- Identifying and challenging the assumptions that underlie ideas.
- Examining the evidence for knowledge and ideas.
- Recognising the role of feelings when working with ideas.
- Being able to use ideas and to make an argument and an informed judgement.
- Taking a critical stance towards your own process of thinking. This is one aspect of **metacognition**, which we will deal with in more depth in Chapter 10.
  (Barnett, 1994; Cottrell, 2011; Moon, 2005, 2008; Redmond, 2006)

You will find that the term 'analysis' is often combined with the term 'critical'. Below is a definition of analysis.

Concept summary: Analysis

Analysis involves:

- examining in detail the different aspects of an issue;
- looking at something from different perspectives;
- breaking something into its component parts.

You will see that there is some overlap between the terms – both involve looking at an issue in depth and detail; both require you to use different perspectives to consider an issue. Analysis also involves breaking something into its elements or constituent parts. When thinking critically, analytic skills will be necessary; however, because critical thinking includes many more thought processes, you need to go beyond analysis.

Case study: analysing a video clip

On Linda's course, the students were shown a short video clip from an NMC video on safeguarding:

www.youtube.com/watch?v=WgWbPK1L_v0&lr=1&uid=-qjEgoAtk9Hvi8z65sIk3Q

The midwifery excerpt is of a busy clinic scene showing a midwife not fully engaging with a woman whose first language is not English. Instead, she communicates predominantly with the woman's partner. The midwife appears to miss obvious signs of domestic abuse. After watching the video the students were asked to work in groups to write an analysis of the episode of care.

One group wrote a short description of what had happened:

> The midwife communicated more with the woman's partner; she did not suggest using a translator. She chatted with the man, and in general she just carried on with her tasks and did not take the opportunity to talk directly to the woman, make eye contact with her or ask her about her needs or concerns. She missed both subtle and obvious clues that might have suggested domestic abuse.

One group formed a judgement, not based on evidence, and wrote the following:

> The midwife spent far too much time in an inappropriate bantering dialogue with the man. She didn't even introduce herself. The man was obviously dominating the whole scenario. The midwife could have put the woman at risk if she put a foot wrong, but she could have been more challenging.

The tutor, Jean, encouraged the group to be more analytic. She asked them to consider the following.

- *The verbal communication used by the midwife, the woman and her partner; the words and expressions used and the explicit and implicit messages conveyed by them.*
- *The pace of the interaction.*
- *The non-verbal communication – the body language, the expression on their faces, where the midwife placed herself, how she set the tone of the clinic appointment and conducted the whole episode of care.*
- *What it might have felt like to be the midwife in that situation – what was she trying to achieve?*
- *What reasons there might be for the midwife avoiding the woman.*
- *What it might have felt like to have been the woman.*
- *Why the man behaved in the way that he did.*
- *The four phases of the interaction: the introduction; the focus on the task; the uncovering of the injury; and the midwife's response. What happened in each phase? What could have been done differently? What should the midwife have done?*

continued . . .

> By using these questions, Jean encouraged the students to break the interaction between the midwife and the couple into component parts and hence be more analytical. This enabled the students to think much more carefully and to identify how it could have been handled differently. Jean asked the students to read about communication (Bach and Grant, 2011) before the next session so that this analysis could be linked to theories.

Developing as a critical thinker

Activity 5.1   *Reflection*

Areas for development

Read carefully the list of aspects of critical thinking above. Write down the ways in which your thinking will need to develop in order for you to become a critical thinker.

Comment

Below you will find some ways of developing critical thinking, illustrated with some case studies of students.

Knowing when critical thinking is needed

It will be important to appreciate when assignment titles and marking criteria are specifically requiring critical thought. When this is the case you will usually find the adjective *critically* in front of a verb, for example:

- critically analyse;
- critically investigate;
- critically evaluate;
- critically explore.

However, beyond the first year of the degree, critical thinking is routinely expected. It should be an integral part of the way you think and approach your studies – not just when it is included in the assignment or essay title.

Taking a different approach to learning

You will need to develop a deep rather than surface approach to learning (Moon, 2005). Thompson (2000) notes that an important part of critical thinking is not being reductionist – students must explore the complexity and many sides of an issue rather than reducing it to a single explanation. Taking a deep approach to learning will enable you to avoid taking issues at face value and help you to identify and challenge the (often hidden) assumptions behind arguments. In Chapter 1 we considered deep, surface and strategic approaches and noted their characteristics. We also noted that they are not fixed and that students can develop approaches that are more conducive to learning (Entwistle et al., 2001; Moon, 2008).

Understanding the academic use of critical

In the academic world taking a critical stance does not carry the negative meaning that some people might assume.

Case study: Linda seeks clarification

When she saw the term critically *in an assignment guideline, Linda realised she felt slightly uncomfortable. Similarly, when she saw the term* argument *she was a little uneasy. She talked to her tutor, Suranne, about this and was reassured to hear that this is not an uncommon response and that women, in particular, sometimes find it hard to challenge in their academic work.*

Linda also thought about her experience as a busy nurse dealing with complex changes and what sometimes felt like constant demands for efficiency; being seen as challenging things at work was viewed negatively, and there was often a pressure to conform and 'get on with it'.

Suranne clarified that in the academic world, to be critical is essential. It does not mean being harsh or unpleasant; instead it is about the careful examination of ideas in order to put together a reasoned and well-thought-out piece of work.

Making an argument is not necessarily about disagreement but about using reason and evidence to support a particular point of view.

Becoming an active learner

You will need to develop your capacity to become an active learner. In critical thinking you are learning to learn as well as learning about midwifery. However, students sometimes start with what Freire (1972) called the banking concept of learning. They envisage that knowledgeable, powerful tutors will fill them up with what they need to know, providing the answers to all their questions. This view is sometimes held because of students' experiences of school where they were expected to be passive learners. If this was the case for you, you may find it a struggle to move to becoming an active learner – discovering things for yourself and creating new ideas.

Case study: Maggie and the banking model

Linda's friend Maggie tended to adopt the banking model of learning. She was keen to get her qualification and wanted her tutors to tell her exactly *what she needed to know so she could get on with things and feel more in control. She and Linda had discussed how they had found it hard to be learners again at university and in clinical practice, but Maggie was finding it even more difficult, and at one point was considering giving up the*

---

continued . . . •••

course, so Linda encouraged her to see her course tutor. Maggie found it a relief to talk about her feelings of annoyance and frustration. The tutor suggested that it might be helpful to do some learning about learning, and together they identified some activities Maggie could work on: slowing down; reflecting; exploring assumptions; trying to think of alternative ways of thinking; looking out for connections between her knowledge and new material. Maggie did not find this easy, but because her motivation to be a midwife was strong, and because she had Linda's support, she was able to persevere with it.

Critical thinking is a deeper, more complex way of thinking. Like Maggie you may need to be self-aware, examine yourself and go through some struggles in order to move to a more active way of learning.

Nervousness about making judgements

Students can be anxious about their ability – or even their right – to make judgements about theories and ideas.

Case study: Nazneen finds out about making judgements

Nazneen had read an article about the reorganisation of postnatal care and was finding it hard to use the piece in her assignment. She had read and re-read the article but could not find a reference to any attempt to ascertain women's views in the discussion on the development of postnatal clinics and the changes in the pattern of home visiting. She was surprised to think that she had identified what seemed to be a gap in the literature on this, and she did not know how to approach this in her essay. She discussed this with her tutor Ifor, who was very positive about her noticing this omission and confirmed that it is an accepted part of being an academic thinker and writer that your ideas will be challenged, critiqued, explored and developed. In academic work, making a judgement is not a negative comment on someone's writing but rather a reasoned conclusion based on weighing up positives and negatives. Nazneen was aware that Ifor had been a major contributor to a midwifery textbook, but she was interested to hear that he had revised some of the work in the second edition because of the feedback from students on the midwifery course who had used the text.

Seeing the relevance to midwifery practice

Some students might find it difficult to see the relevance of critical thinking for a degree in midwifery, which is often thought of as involving getting on and doing things with no need for deep thinking. However, thinking skills are transferable to the practice of midwifery. Practitioners are required, on a daily basis, to make decisions about complex issues, most of which will not have a single correct answer. Midwives must be able to consider the possible options based on an analysis of the impact of different approaches. They need to weigh evidence, examine arguments and understand and demonstrate the thinking and reasoning underlying their decisions. Critical thinking will help them do this and is the basis and foundation of thoughtful resolution of issues and effective practice. Moon (2005) notes that students on placements have a real opportunity to use their critical thinking skills through making judgments and decisions about live issues. This is why, on your course, as well as using these skills to consider theories and approaches, you may be asked to critically analyse case studies or incidents from practice.

In Chapter 7 we will be considering reflective thinking and practice. Here it is worth noting that there is a strong link between reflective thinking and critical thinking. While reflection tends to be more about one's own self, experiences and feelings, reflective activities can support critical thinking.

The stages in critical thinking

It can be helpful when considering a complex process such as critical thinking to separate it into stages. Again we have synthesised ideas from writers on the subject.

Critical thinking includes: identifying a range of positions, arguments and conclusions; evaluating the evidence for alternative points of view; and weighing up opposing arguments. We began to do this in a descriptive way in Chapter 4 when considering Linda's assignment. However, critical thinking is broader and deeper. In particular, it extends and amplifies the ways in which students should evaluate ideas. This includes the following aspects.

- Exploring the history of the ideas and **principles** under consideration.
- Reading between the lines, identifying the assumptions and value positions behind the thinking. In midwifery this could mean utilising professional values.
- Developing a sound understanding of the sources of evidence for the ideas and evaluating them; appreciating the difference between primary and secondary sources.
- Thinking about the limitations of the ideas; searching for flaws and weaknesses in the arguments. This requires a realisation and understanding that all knowledge is contested, challengeable and open to debate.
- Reflecting on issues in a structured way; thinking about why, emotionally, some ideas might be more appealing than others.
- Making judgements and drawing conclusions, based on all of the above, about the validity of the idea, using the best evidence.
- Putting forward your own proposition, while recognising its limited nature, in a structured, clear and well-reasoned way.
  (Barnett, 1994; Cottrell, 2011; Moon, 2005).

Using critical thinking

Case study: Paul's assignment

Below is an assignment requiring critical thinking that Paul's group was given:

Understanding domestic abuse is an essential component of good midwifery practice. Critically discuss this statement.

In order to develop his ability to critically analyse, Paul first considered and noted what he might need to consider under each aspect of critical thinking listed above.

Comment

Below are Paul's answers. They illustrate the processes of critical thinking. The length of Paul's assignment was constrained by the required word count. However, it assisted his development as a critical thinker to explore sources and ideas broadly and in depth before writing his assignment.

Identifying a range of positions, arguments and conclusions

Paul identified several different perspectives on domestic abuse and its significance in midwifery practice. In order to do this he explored a range of positions on the definition, causes and impact of domestic abuse. He used standard textbooks dealing with theories from sociology and psychology, as well as material covering legal and social policy perspectives. In order to evaluate the evidence supporting different arguments he considered research articles, and current and historical statistics on domestic abuse, together with policy documents and some specialist websites.

In his search for relevant literature Paul also thought about groups who have traditionally been marginalised – for example, people from Black and Minority Ethnic (BME) communities, and disabled people. Because the title asked him to think about domestic abuse and midwifery, he also explored material that discussed the importance of domestic abuse in midwifery practice. This search revealed gaps – for example, midwifery books that did not make the connection between domestic abuse and child protection. He realised that sometimes what is not mentioned can be as important as what is.

Exploring the history of the ideas and principles under consideration

Here Paul explored how ideas about domestic abuse, including its significance for midwifery practice, have developed historically. This included:

- the lack of public attention before the 1970s;
- the factors in the development of understanding in the 1970s;
- current definitions;
- historical and current theories on causes;
- statistics on its extent;
- midwifery's historical and current response to domestic abuse.

Through using this approach to considering ideas about domestic abuse and midwifery Paul realised that knowledge is not absolute: it is constructed – it shifts and changes.

Reading between the lines, identifying the assumptions and value positions behind the thinking, including consideration of the NMC code (NMC, 2008)

Here Paul considered the values reflected in different understandings of domestic abuse. This included:

- the values implicit in the use of the term domestic abuse;
- the assumptions that lie behind the view that domestic abuse is a private matter to be sorted out within the family;

- the feminist writers of the 1970s and 1980s who rejected traditional individualistic explanations of domestic abuse and instead focused on theories of patriarchy;
- the values that underlie midwifery's current public health focus on domestic abuse.

Developing a sound understanding of the sources of evidence for the ideas and evaluating them; appreciating the difference between primary and secondary sources

In order to examine the different sides of an argument Paul needed to know where to access the evidence that might either support or dispute that position. This included accessing valid and relevant sources of material, as discussed earlier. To achieve this he required a good appreciation of the range of sources available and the ability to select appropriately. His course handbooks included really helpful reading lists, but he also tried to delve deeper and found it particularly useful to examine the references upon which the authors he was reading had drawn.

Primary, or original, sources are those produced or published at the time of the events under consideration. For this assignment these might be:

- books from the 1970s that were written to convey the emerging feminist analysis of domestic violence;
- contemporary accounts of people's experience of how midwives responded to domestic abuse;
- midwifery textbooks written several decades ago;
- the data from research on domestic abuse and midwifery;
- policy documents from relevant periods.

Secondary sources are materials written or produced about the issue, usually some time later. For this assignment these might be:

- current documents about the setting up of the first women's refuges;
- reports of research studies on domestic abuse and midwifery;
- books, articles and web pages about domestic abuse.

At this stage of his studies Paul focused mostly on secondary sources. However, he was aware that some books, known as seminal texts, provided such new and original thinking that they continue to play an important role in the understanding of the subject. Paul looked forward to using primary sources in his **dissertation**. For this assignment he looked at one example:

Dobash, R and Dobash, R (1980) *Violence against wives: a case against the patriarchy*. Shepton Mallet: Open Books.

This book is an account of research into violence towards wives carried out in Scotland in the 1970s. Based on their research Dobash and Dobash (1980) argue that the patriarchal family system where the husband's authority creates a subordinate position for women is fundamental to understanding violence to wives. They found that many incidents of abuse arose from arguments about money, housework or childcare, and that men asserted their authority and power through the use of violence.

Evaluating the sources will also mean considering the usefulness of the source of evidence. You could ask the following questions.

- What is its relevance?
- Does it provide a useful theoretical perspective?
- Does this help me to open up the debate or does it close it down?
- Was this an important contribution to changing the way domestic violence and abuse was understood?

Thinking about the limitations of the ideas; searching for flaws and weaknesses in the arguments. This requires a realisation and understanding that all knowledge is contested, challengeable and open to debate

Through his exploration of the history and range of ideas about domestic abuse Paul came to appreciate that there have been, and still are, different views. Moving on from grasping the ideas, Paul, recognising that all knowledge must be open to scrutiny, explored their limitations. He used the list suggested for evaluating that is set out in Chapter 4.

- What are the strengths/positives?
- Why are these strengths?
- What are the limitations/weaknesses?
- Why are these weaknesses?
- What was not covered? What gaps are there?
- What aspects of social inclusion were considered?
- What aspects of social inclusion were not taken into account?
- Were the values of midwifery integrated?

Reflecting on issues in a structured way; thinking about why emotionally some ideas might be more appealing than others

Here Paul needed to think about how his own experiences or lack of personal knowledge of domestic abuse might leave him more sympathetic to one view rather than another. For example, he felt very drawn to research evidence that suggested that midwives identified a number of obstacles to routinely asking women if they have experienced domestic abuse. Paul had observed this at an antenatal clinic and had been reflecting on it. But he was resistant to some arguments because they reminded him of some issues that he had not previously considered and made him a bit uncomfortable. This was the case when he found research about the lack of help offered to women from BME communities who reported domestic abuse. It alerted him to an area of practice he had not really considered before. Paul learnt that it was important to consider and articulate why some ideas and theories are more attractive to you than others.

Making judgements and drawing conclusions, based on all of the above, about the validity of the idea, using the best evidence

At this stage Paul needed to systematically pull together all the ideas that he had previously explored – their strengths and their weaknesses. His judgements about these led to his conclusions. In this assignment Paul needed to keep a clear focus on the assignment statement – *Understanding domestic abuse is an essential component of good midwifery practice* – so he needed to conclude whether the statement was valid and give his reasons for his assertion. Having examined all the evidence, he concluded that for good midwifery practice having an understanding of domestic abuse is necessary, but not sufficient, as understanding should lead to changes in the way midwives work with women and their families.

Putting forward your own proposition, while recognising its limited nature, in a structured, clear and well-reasoned way

Finally, as a critically thinking student midwife, following on from his conclusions Paul put forward his own thoughts on the issue, which included some ways in which midwives' under-standing might be translated into action. So he suggested the following.

- Midwives could support each other if they found it difficult to ask questions about domestic abuse.
- Midwives could seek the support of supervisors of midwives or draw on the expertise of public health midwives, consultant midwives or other local specialists in the health and social care teams.
- Local training and input from local specialist public health midwives could update midwives on the latest research in relation to women from BME communities and develop awareness and debate about good practice.

Paul's proposals related back to, and followed logically from, the arguments made in the assignment.

In this example we have not considered how Paul might structure his assignment. Rather, we have shown how Paul used the framework for critical thinking to work on his assignment.

The characteristics of critical thinkers

Activity 5.2   *Critical thinking*

Critical thinkers

Given what you have now learnt about critical thinking, make a list of the attributes of student midwives who are critical thinkers.

Comment

You might have come up with some of the following.

- An enquiring and curious mind.
- Intellectual honesty.
- Well read, with a good background knowledge of midwifery in its broad context.
- Open-mindedness.
- Intelligent scepticism or polite doubt – in *The Victoria Climbié Enquiry* Lord Laming (2003, p205) called this *respectful uncertainty*.
- The ability to think in a systematic way.
- The ability to differentiate writing that sets out arguments from other types of writing.
- Self-knowledge – being aware why we might prefer one explanation to another.
- Open to challenge: ready to have long-held assumptions challenged.
- Being prepared to move beyond the comfort zone of what you know.
- Brave enough to take some risks.
- The capacity to use support to develop the confidence necessary for forming your own viewpoint.
  (Barnett, 1994; Cottrell, 2011; Moon, 2005, 2008)

Activity 5.3   *Reflection*

Self-evaluation

Take some time to consider which of these attributes of a critically thinking midwifery student you possess and which you need to develop.

Comment

This is, of course, a formidable list – one to aim for, not where you would expect to be at this stage. It is worth noting that the list includes *affective* or emotional qualities in addition to *cognitive* or thinking attributes.

Using critical thinking to explore a situation from practice

During your course you will be expected to apply your critical thinking and analytical skills to case studies and incidents from practice. This will entail using the theories, knowledge and understanding you have developed as tools to make sense of a situation and inform your midwifery practice.

> ## Case study
>
> *Nazneen had the opportunity to observe a planned home birth with her mentor Sandy. The expectant mother Denise placed a lot of importance on being in her own house and having her family around her during the birth, including her partner Tom, their three children aged six, four and two years, her father and her stepmother. After the birth of her last child Denise had had a post-partum haemorrhage. Sandy has some concerns about the plans for a home birth and has discussed carefully with Denise and Tom the options and the risks.*
>
> *Sandy asked Nazneen to identify the theories and research she would use to help analyse the situation and formulate pragmatic plans if she was a qualified midwife.*

Comment

Nazneen identified the following.

- To explore the concerns and risks for Denise – research relating to both post-partum haemorrhage and place of birth.
- To appreciate Denise's strong wish to have her family members around her during the birth – theories about the sociology of the family.
- To think about the potential impact on the younger children of the birth and any birth complications – theories from psychology concerning child development.
- To understand Sandy's intervention – theories about communication from counselling and psychology.

Nazneen was aware that, when she wrote this up in her portfolio, she would need to apply a critical perspective to each of these areas of knowledge.

Critical writing skills

Using critical writing skills should assist you in conveying your thoughts and ideas. Critical writing should:

- contain only essential descriptive writing;
- be clear and precise;
- present arguments in a consistent way;
- indicate the relevance of the material included;
- be carefully selective about the amount of detail required;
- give reasons for the selection of information;
- show how ideas or arguments are connected;
- structure information in order of importance;
- show how different arguments or ideas are connected;
- use language effectively to convey arguments and ideas;
- signpost the reader through the argument through skilful use of language;

- make a reasoned judgement;
- reach a logical conclusion based on arguments.
  (Cottrell, 2011; Moon, 2005)

Activity 5.4   *Critical thinking*

Different kinds of writing

Compare the list above with the outline of descriptive language in Chapter 4. Identify the differences between the two types of language.

An example of critically analytic writing can be found in Chapter 9 (pages 130–4) where Paul is critically analysing research on stillbirth.

Chapter summary

In this chapter we have identified what being a critical thinker means, the important characteristics and ways of developing these attributes. We have looked at ways this thinking might be used in assignments and in practice, and noted the features of critical writing. It is not possible to become a critical thinker and writer simply by reading this chapter. It will be part of your development as a learner, both in university and when on practice placements. By the end of the course you should be demonstrating these skills, as you will require them both in your studies and when you become a professional midwife. This links us to the next chapter, in which we explore how you can use your university learning during your practice placement.

Further reading

Bach, S and Grant, A (2011) *Communication and interpersonal skills for nurses* (2nd edition). Exeter: Learning Matters.

A good grounding in communication and interpersonal skills for student health professionals.

Cottrell, S (2011) *Critical thinking skills* (2nd edition). Basingstoke: Palgrave Macmillan.

A comprehensive guide to developing effective analysis and argument, written for a general audience; contains many useful activities.

Price, B and Harrington, A (2013) *Critical thinking and writing for nursing students*. London: Learning Matters/Sage.

A useful introduction to the subject – aimed primarily at nurses but much of the content is equally applicable to midwives.

Chapter 6
Applying university learning on your practice placements

This chapter will help you to meet the Quality Assurance Agency for Higher Education (2008) requirement that students studying at Level 5 are able to:

- demonstrate ability to apply underlying concepts and principles outside the context in which they were first studied, including, where appropriate, the applications of those principles in an employment context.

NMC Standards for Pre-registration Midwifery Education

This chapter will address the following competencies:

Domain: Effective midwifery practice
Determine and provide programmes of care and support for women which:

- are appropriate to the needs, contexts, culture and choices of women, babies and their families;
- are based on best evidence and clinical judgement.

Provide seamless care and, where appropriate, interventions, in partnership with women and other care providers during the antenatal period which:

- are appropriate for women's assessed needs, context and culture;
- are evidence based.

Work in partnership with women and other care providers during the postnatal period to provide seamless care and interventions which:

- are appropriate to the woman's assessed needs, context and culture;
- are evidence based.

Care for and monitor women during the puerperium, offering the necessary evidence-based advice and support regarding the baby and self-care.

Domain: Achieving quality care through evaluation and research
Apply relevant knowledge to the midwife's own practice in structured ways which are capable of evaluation.

> **Chapter aims**
>
> After reading this chapter you should be able to:
>
> - see the links between your university learning and your experiences during practice learning;
> - apply theories relevant to midwifery to your practice.

Introduction

We have previously acknowledged the applied nature of midwifery knowledge and the importance of making connections between university learning and midwifery practice. By this stage in your midwifery degree, you are expected to be able to apply your academic learning in other contexts. This means applying theories and principles when you are on your practice placement. The purpose of this chapter is to help you to be able to make these connections between theoretical knowledge learnt in university and the world of midwifery.

> **Activity 6.1**   *Reflection*
>
> **Reflecting on placements**
>
> Think about your experience of practice on placement and identify any difficulties you have faced relating university work to placement experiences.

Comment

Several factors can militate against the application of theories, concepts and principles. Using knowledge when in university to work on case studies is valuable, providing a safe space to test out ideas and learn from errors. But it can seem a world away from the reality of practice, where students experience the pressure of needing to provide answers, to make decisions and to perform effectively. The pace of activity on placement may suggest that there simply is not enough time to give attention to high-level thought – it being more important to get on and do the work. Students also face the demands of learning to become competent midwives while under the spotlight of assessment in practice. They may feel that building their skills and getting on with completing their practice learning portfolio should take priority.

You will find, however, that providing the evidence of your competence cannot be separated from your use of theoretical knowledge. In order to meet a satisfactory level of competence, you need to articulate the thinking behind your actions. Bringing together practice and theory may be hard work. However, your goal, by the end of your degree, should be what Secker (1993) called a 'fluent approach' to practice. This means being able to choose and apply relevant knowledge and combine smoothly different sources of understanding from both theory and personal and professional experience.

Applying knowledge

To apply knowledge means to be able to put it into operation in order to help you to organise and make sense of your experiences. You should be able to use what you have learnt in university to enhance your learning during your placement. Macaulay (2000) describes this as the transfer of learning that occurs whenever existing knowledge, abilities and skills – what you already know and can do – affect the learning or performance of new tasks, or understanding and practising in a new situation. This will necessitate questioning and thinking critically (Carr, 1995). At this level of an undergraduate degree it means having *understanding of the need to select principles and facts appropriate to the problem in hand* and being able to *apply the principles* (Lyons and Bennett, 2001, p180). For midwives this means using relevant knowledge to guide practice.

There are different educational theories used to understand this application of knowledge. Eraut (1994) outlines two different kinds of professional knowledge – propositional and process.

• Propositional knowledge consists of theories and concepts and principles that can be used in different ways; replication, application, interpretation or association.
• Process knowledge involves the application of propositional knowledge, shifting your thinking from knowing *that* to knowing *how*.

The application of knowledge, with which we are concerned in this chapter, in practice involves both seeing the connections between theory and practice, and using the knowledge effectively.

Another way of looking at the application of knowledge is to consider Kolb's learning cycle, which is a model or theory about how people learn (see Figure 6.1). It suggests that from concrete

4. Application of the concepts
to new experience
(Active experimentation)

1. Experience on
placement
(Concrete experience)

3. Theories, principles and
concepts of midwifery
(Abstract conceptualisation)

2. Thoughts and
reflection
(Reflective observation)

Figure 6.1 Kolb's cycle of learning

Source: Adapted from Parker (2010) and first published in this form in Walker (2011).

experiences (1), such as direct practical experience on placement, learners move to abstract conceptualisation, or theories and principles (3), through thought and reflection (2). This enables theories and concepts to be applied in new situations, also known as active experimentation (4). The cycle then continues as this experimentation leads to new concrete experiences – and the process carries on. This model helps us to understand how the application of theory to real practice experience might occur: through reflection on the experience and experimentation or trying out the concepts in relation to practice. Learning, therefore, is an ongoing continuous process.

When using the model you can either start with your experiences or with theories. If you begin with your placement experiences, you apply thought and reflection to them in order to move, through the cycle, to the theories and principles that might help you to make sense of it. You then apply the theories to new situations, showing how you have learned to use theory in practice. Alternatively, you might start with theories and move round the cycle from there. What is important is that you will need to use and build on existing concepts. It is worth noting that simply having experiences does not lead to learning; you have to actively work with them using reflection and thought in order to develop. In this way you will be moving backwards and forwards between theory and practice (Parker, 2010; Thompson, 2000). In Chapter 7 we will look in more detail at the process of reflection, which is an important way of thinking about your experiences.

Activity 6.2   *Reflection*

Relating theory to practice on your placement

Think about and write down:

- what you would find helpful from the placement to assist you in relating theory to practice;
- what you can do to assist the process of relating theory to practice.

Research summary: learning from placements

Research from general and midwifery education research suggests the following answers.

A helpful placement will offer you:

- the opportunity to have experiences that will support your learning;
- a practice midwife mentor with whom you have a trusting relationship and who allows you to learn from your mistakes;
- a practice mentor who can draw your attention to the potential for transfer of learning and help you make connections;
- a mentor who is a helpful role model;
- a culture supportive of applying university learning to practice;

- a shared language about learning;
- space to think.

You will find it easier to relate theory to practice if you are able to:

- organise your thinking in ways that help you to recognise meaningful patterns and principles;
- secure a sound grasp of university learning;
- critically analyse;
- learn from experience;
- actively think about your experience;
- make a deliberate effort to relate the new experience to concepts you already possess;
- be a motivated learner.
  (Armstrong, 2008; Lister, 2000; Macaulay, 2000; Miles, 2008)

Writing about practice

On your course you will be required to write about your practice both in your PDP or portfolio of practice learning and in university assignments. While in some academic work it is not seen as appropriate to use the first person – or 'I' – in essays and assignments, in midwifery it can be acceptable. In our experience the use of 'I' enables students to more clearly outline and analyse their practice in addition to explaining their thinking and reasoning. However, you should always check this with your tutors and exercise care not to overuse personal pronouns.

When demonstrating your ability to apply theory and knowledge to placement experiences it will be essential to keep the two components woven together in your writing. There is a risk of including a paragraph on practice followed by a paragraph on theory, but writing in this way will not show that you can make and articulate the connections. Howarth (1999, p327) notes that the portfolio *provides the ideal opportunity to unite the theory and practice of midwifery*, and you should aim for this connection in your writing.

Theories and practice

In Chapter 3 we noted that midwifery draws on theories concerning:

- the physiology and psychology of maternity and childbirth;
- ways of going about midwifery most effectively;
- the organisations within which midwives work;
- the lives of the women they are working with, including their internal (psychological) world and their external (social) world.

Here you are asked to apply in practice theories you have learnt in university about aspects of the world of the people who use the service. On your placement you will regularly observe issues that impact on the ways women experience their births and pregnancies, and manage afterwards. You will also come across issues that affect midwifery practice.

You may feel very strongly about what you experience – from pleasure and admiration to sadness, anger and concern. It is important to analyse your response and learn from this. This can help you to move on from, and beyond, these observations and feelings to a conceptual and theoretical appreciation of the relevant laws and social policies that frame people's lives and how midwifery services are provided. You should, in your thinking, be able to move from concrete situations and experiences to a grasp of policies and theoretical principles underpinning them.

Case study: using social policy

Paul was observing his mentor in an antenatal clinic; specifically focusing his attention on parents attending a clinic for the first time in pregnancy at eleven weeks, he was keeping a diary of his experience and observations. Below is what he wrote:

> Today I joined Dilys who was 'booking in' Samira, a mother from Algeria. I noticed that there were some specific questions on the booking-in form about diet, smoking, drinking, domestic abuse and BCG immunisations. Dilys paid particular attention to these questions and took the time to make sure that Samira understood what she was saying. This took a while as Samira has difficulty grasping some English words at first but Dilys was very patient and put a lot of emphasis on this part of the meeting. Afterwards I asked Dilys about this and she talked about the increasing focus for midwives on public health issues. I had written an essay about domestic abuse and, in my reading for that had come across references to midwives' public health role. I started thinking about the different roles midwives can take on and how this had developed.

Most of this diary entry consists of descriptive writing outlining some aspects of Paul's observation. However, you can also see that he has started to think and reflect – to process – what he saw. He has wondered about the contribution midwives might be able to make to the health of the community.

Paul continued to think about this and wonder where the thinking behind this had come from. He recalled some of the lectures in university that discussed health policies. He already knew that everyday midwifery practice is shaped by broader social and political thinking, but his recent experiences were now making this understanding come to life.

He went back to his notes, handouts, books and other literature and read about:

- *the early development of public health in the 1870s;*
- *the impact public health measures have had on improving the life chances of the population;*
- *the development of the public health role for midwives;*
- *the continuing and expanding health promotion role of midwives;*
- *how decisions have been made about the public health issues midwives should focus on;*
- *the impact on the working lives of midwives.*

Paul had appropriately selected pre-existing knowledge and developed his understanding through placement observation and using social policy theory in practice.

Activity 6.3   *Critical thinking*

The social context of your placement

Think about the day-to-day lives and experiences of the women who use midwifery services. Identify the legislation and social policies that form the context of their lives.

Comment

Shardlow (2007) suggests the following approaches to social policy are relevant to those providing public services.

- The *values or principles* that might underlie social policy such as equality, social need and rights.
- The *politics* of social policy; for example, modernisation, the mixed economy of care and deregulation.
- The *content* of social policy in five major areas of importance: education, health, housing, social care and social security. In turn these could be considered under headings such as social issues, social problems and the experiences of groups.

It might be useful to see where your answer fits into Shardlow's approaches.

Theories of how to do midwifery

We will now focus on how you can use what you have learnt in university to think about planning care with women and families.

When in university, despite using case studies, video clips and role play to explore different ways of working, students can find it a challenge to think about their application in practice. When you are on placement you will need to make these connections.

Case study: Tara

As part of her caseload at the end of her second year Nazneen is supporting Tara through her pregnancy. Tara is 17 and lives with her mother. She is now 30 weeks pregnant, and although her health appears good, there are concerns about the baby's growth. Tara had booked late at 20 weeks and did not attend her last clinic appointment. She says she smokes 15 cigarettes a day and has told Nazneen that she sometimes forgets to eat.

Nazneen's first approach had been to follow local guidelines to refer Tara to resources thought to be helpful – the teenage support group and the smoking cessation link worker for maternity services. However, Tara had reacted in quite a hostile fashion to these plans. She said she had had a friend who had not liked the teenage support group coordinator and that she was not interested in talking to anyone else about smoking.

Nazneen thought over what she had learnt in university about young mothers and some of the reasons they might be resistant. She wondered if Tara felt as if she was being told what to do and where to go. Nazneen's

---

continued . . .

thinking also took into account the need to ensure the safety of Tara's baby, and she recognised the importance of local guidelines relating to fetal growth. One university seminar that had particularly interested her outlined a partnership approach in midwifery. When on placement she had mentioned this to her new community midwife mentor, Natalie, and learnt that Natalie had used this approach in New Zealand. There the partnership approach has been built into legislation and the funding structure for the whole of the maternity services. Nazneen liked the principles of the partnership approach: women-centred; collaborative planning; continuity; being 'with-women'; choice and control; self-determination (Carolan and Hodnett, 2007; Mander, 2011). It all sounded good in theory, but Nazneen was not confident about how she might put it into practice.

She shared with Natalie her frustration at not being able to make progress with Tara, explained that she wanted to rethink how she was working with her, and tentatively suggested the possibility of using a partnership approach. Natalie asked Nazneen what she felt Tara needed and what would be welcomed by her. Together they agreed that a partnership approach might be helpful to Tara. Natalie recommended more reading, which strengthened Nazneen's understanding. Nazneen realised that her plan to text Tara about her next appointment had been a good start in moving towards partnership working using the principle of being 'with-women' and understanding what was important and meaningful in their lives.

The next appointment with Tara took place in the local children's centre. Nazneen had phoned Tara with various suggestions about where to meet and given the choice to Tara. Nazneen made sure that she listened carefully to Tara so she could appreciate what might be going on for her and what her anxieties might be. She learnt that Tara thought that being referred meant she was being passed on to another midwife and would not be part of Nazneen's caseload. After some discussion and reassurance Tara agreed to meet with the teenage support worker along with Nazneen. Gradually Tara relaxed and seemed pleased with information Nazneen gave her about the support group and the activities young mothers did there. Tara opened up about some of her worries – above all, she seemed to fear not being listened to and being judged. It became clear that Tara had been given mixed messages by friends and family about pregnancy and childbirth and their opinions of Tara as a mother. This had knocked her confidence. In addition she had recently ended her relationship with Ben, the baby's father, hated 'getting fat', and was fearful of the baby being big. Concerns about money were very real for her and her own mother. Nazneen worked hard to keep her attention on what Tara was sharing so she could be truly alongside her and 'with-woman'. She felt she had been able to learn more about Tara's individual fears and hopes. This enabled her to make some suggestions that Tara seemed to be happy with. Although Tara remained reluctant to see the smoking cessation worker, she liked the idea of downloading some apps on her phone – one that might help her to think about quitting and another that gave her day-to-day information about her growing baby.

Over the next few weeks Nazneen continued to listen carefully to Tara, and together they planned for the rest of the pregnancy and for the birth. Tara did not miss any more appointments and kept in close contact by text. Nazneen worked hard to remember the principles of collaborative planning and to avoid the stance of professionals always knowing what is best. Wherever possible, she encouraged Tara to make her own decisions. Tara had chosen her mother as her birth companion, and they had both enjoyed designing Tara's 'birth-plan T-shirt' – an activity in the teenage support group programme. Throughout, Natalie ensured that Nazneen's records were of a good standard and that the plan of care did not present avoidable risks.

Concerns about the baby's growth diminished, and Tara decided to have her baby in the local midwifery-led unit. She had talked about her anxieties for the birth both with Nazneen and with the group. At first she thought she wanted an epidural, as her friend had said how great they were. Then she looked at some birth films

continued . . .

suggested by the teenage support worker and read information on a blog site from young women who had given birth in a pool, and she become very interested in water birth. She seemed embarrassed about the prospect of giving birth naked, but when Nazneen suggested she could wear the birth plan T-shirt she felt reassured. On the night of the birth, Natalie was not available to attend. However, Emma, the birth centre midwife on shift was kind and careful, and both Nazneen and Tara felt very well supported. Emma was interested in how Nazneen had planned the care and worked with Tara and asked for ideas for reading about partnership working. Tara gave birth to a 7lb boy, Alfie, in the pool in her T-shirt.

Learning from practice experience

Nazneen was able to identify a number of learning points that she thought would guide and inform her in future experiences of midwifery.

- By active listening, Nazneen had opened the door for Tara to share her views and fears. She learnt about Tara's motivation and feelings and how she was trying to protect herself by sticking to her own certainties
- Tara's main concerns about the pregnancy were not the same as those identified by Nazneen at their first meeting. It had been important to refocus and try to appreciate what was important for Tara. Adopting a woman-centred approach to planning care was initially slightly uncomfortable for Nazneen and she had to think carefully about this.
- She had learnt quickly that her role was to enable Tara to find a way forward, not to do everything for her. Nazneen liked the images of a signpost or a bridge as symbols of midwifery care and now found these useful to visualise before she started talking to women.
- Supporting Tara's confidence in her ability to make decisions about her care, her birth and her baby appeared to strengthen her as a mother, and to strengthen her relationship with her own mother and the rest of her support network.

It can be helpful, when developing your learning skills to have an awareness of the learning process and what supports it. Appreciating how you have learnt and developed is a step towards becoming a more autonomous, self-directing student. We will discuss this further in Chapter 10. Below is an activity that explores how Nazneen developed her learning.

Activity 6.4   *Critical thinking*

Nazneen's learning

Look back at the learning processes Nazneen went through and identify the ways in which she was able to relate theory to practice.

Comment

We can look at this in different, yet connected, ways.

- Nazneen was able to select, from what she had learnt at university, an approach to use in practice by recognising the connections between the principles of the approach and Tara's situation and motivation. She developed her understanding of the partnership approach to working and applied it in a thoughtful and careful way considering its usefulness as she proceeded.

- Nazneen began with propositional knowledge (*knowing that* – i.e. what she knew about the theory of the partnership approach). She translated this into process knowledge or *knowing how* the partnership approach could be used in practice.
- Using the Kolb learning cycle model Nazneen began with the theoretical approach (2) that she actively applied (3). From this active experimentation she identified learning that she felt confident she could take to fresh experiences during the course (1).
- In all this Nazneen was supported by her mentor who used questions and discussion to support her in applying this approach in practice.

Other applications of theory

Theories learnt in university can also help us understand dynamics – or what is unconsciously going on – between people. This could be relevant to teams and other working relationships such as supervisor/supervisee or mentor/student, together with interactions between midwives, women and their families. Such issues can evoke strong feelings in people, so using theory to make sense of them can be very helpful.

Activity 6.5 *Decision making*

Applying theory

- Identify one issue in your placement that you have been puzzled by, struggled to make sense of, really enjoyed or found very interesting.
- Think about your 'tool kit' of knowledge.
- Try to identify a theory, concept or principle that you could apply to the issue, deepening your understanding of it.

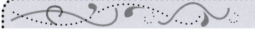

Chapter summary

In this chapter we have focused on how to apply learning in university to the real-life situations you may experience on placement. In order to do this, we have explored some theoretical ideas about learning and begun to consider how an understanding of how we learn can help us grow and develop. However, there are some important issues to which we have given only brief attention – in particular, the importance of reflection. We turn to these in the next and later chapters.

Further reading

Bryar, R and Sinclair, S (eds) (2011) *Theory for midwifery practice* (2nd edition). Basingstoke: Palgrave, Macmillan.

This book both explores the role of theory and provides some examples of its use in midwifery practice.

Chapter 7
Developing as a reflective learner and practitioner

This chapter will help you to meet the Quality Assurance Agency for Higher Education (2008) requirement that students studying at Level 5 are able to:

- demonstrate knowledge and critical understanding of the well-established principles of their area(s) of study and of the ways in which those principles have developed;
- demonstrate ability to apply underlying concepts and principles outside the context in which they were first studied, including, where appropriate, the applications of those principles in an employment context;
- demonstrate knowledge of the main methods of enquiry in the subject(s) relevant to the named award, and ability to evaluate critically the appropriateness of different approaches to solving problems in the field of study;
- demonstrate an understanding of the limits of their knowledge, and how this influences analyses and interpretations based on that knowledge;
- use a range of established techniques to initiate and undertake critical analysis of information, and to propose solutions to problems arising from that analysis.

NMC Standards for Pre-registration Midwifery Education

This chapter will address the following competencies:

Domain: Developing the individual midwife and others
Review, develop and enhance the midwife's own knowledge, skills and fitness to practise. This will include:

- reflecting on the midwife's own practice and making the necessary changes as a result.

Domain: Achieving quality care through evaluation and research
Apply relevant knowledge to the midwife's own practice in structured ways which are capable of evaluation. This will include:

- critical appraisal of the midwife's own practice.

Introduction

The purpose of this chapter is to introduce you to the notion of reflective thinking, an approach to learning that has gained significance in recent years. While it is not included in the generic benchmark statement (QAA, 2008), it is implicit, subsumed in the general academic requirements, since thinking reflectively is a crucial part of thinking critically and effective problem solving (Moon, 2008). The NMC's *Standards for pre-registration midwifery education* (NMC, 2009) require midwives to be able to reflect on their practice and amend how they work as a consequence.

In this chapter we will explore reflective thinking before considering what this means for developing as a reflective midwifery practitioner. The next part of the book will cover the integration of reflective thinking into the repertoire of the student midwife.

What is reflective thinking?

Reflective thinking:

- is the purposeful process of consideration and reconsideration of learning material (knowledge, idea or experiences);
- tends to occur when the learning material is complex or unpredictable;
- involves deep thinking;
- often involves emotions;
- should lead to new understandings.
  (Boud et al., 1985; Moon, 2004).

Thinking back to the previous chapter, you will recall that reflection was one stage in Kolb's cycle of learning, located between concrete experiences and abstract concepts. For Kolb, reflection is a way of thinking that assists the process of making relationships between experiences and theoretical ideas. Schön (1983), a leading writer in this field, pointed out the importance of reflection in the development of knowledge and understanding of professionals. He argued that professional expertise could not rely on the straightforward technical application of theories to problems. Professional practice – especially in work with people – is more complex because it is concerned with uncertain, multi-faceted, real-life situations including value conflicts, so professional artistry based on reflection is needed as well as technical competence. Other writers have taken Schön's ideas and developed them (Boud et al., 1985; Mezirow, 1981).

Boud et al. (1985, p3) define reflective thinking as *those intellectual and affective activities in which individuals engage to explore their experiences in order to lead to new understanding and appreciation.* They see the important ingredients as:

- intellectual activity – thinking;
- affective activity – feeling or experiencing emotions;
- use of these to explore or find out more about experiences, the result of which should be different and fresh thinking.

These are the features of reflective thinking.

- Reflective thinking builds on and develops critical thinking adding other components.
- It requires the deep approach to learning outlined in Chapter 1 because it delves and explores beneath the surface and goes beyond a superficial understanding of issues. It includes not only our experience and practice but also how we have gone about things and the understandings that lie beneath what we have done.
- In exploring beneath the surface, reflective thinking welcomes challenge, doubt, uncertainty and contradictions.
- The professional is an active participant in the use and development of knowledge. So the individual's own experiences and feelings become resources to help develop understanding rather than issues that get in the way of constructing knowledge.
- Reflective thinking can be helped by the learner being exposed to thinking from a different angle or perspective.
- It is aided by developing an understanding and self-awareness of your own learning, or metacognition, an issue we will return to in Chapter 10.
- The new understanding will have an impact on professional practice.
  (Boud et al.,1985; Redmond, 2006; Taylor and White, 2000)

The importance of feelings in reflection

Exploring and attempting to understand one's own feelings are important aspects of reflective thinking. Sometimes reflection may be triggered by uncomfortable feelings (Stuart, 2010). But exploration of one's feelings should routinely be part of reflection because emotion can play an important role in influencing the way in which we experience situations and make sense of them. In reflection we need to learn to be aware of and analyse our feelings. Boud et al. (1985, p26) argue that an important aspect of reflection is *attending to feelings*. By this they mean an exploration of both negative and positive feelings – both those experienced during the incident upon which you are reflecting and those experienced during the reflection. They argue that it may be important to deal with negative feelings that may be obstructing a reflective consideration of events.

Reflection and midwifery practice

Activity 7.1   *Reflection*

The importance of reflective thinking

Think about what is involved in midwifery practice and write down as many reasons as you can why reflective thinking might be important in midwifery education and practice.

Comment

Reflective thinking is seen as particularly important both in midwifery education and training, and in day-to-day practice for a number of reasons. Compare your reasons with the list below.

- Being a midwife means you are involved with aspects of people's lives that have enormous significance: birth, change in life and status and sometimes death. You will often experience strong feelings and be exposed to the emotions of women and families.
- Midwifery is an activity where the reasons for the decisions made about people's lives should be thought out and articulated so that midwives can be held accountable. This is particularly relevant since decisions may be based on particular values or assumptions. Reflective thinking challenges you to look afresh at your value base and ensures you take nothing for granted. Reflective thinking can help to avoid the risk of 'doing midwifery' in a routine way because it helps you to see that each situation has unique aspects to it and that these need to be explored.
- Midwifery is a profession in which the development of practice and learning, during and through experience, is seen as a valuable way of taking forward knowledge and understanding.
- Reflection helps us to move beyond our current frameworks of thinking and opens up ideas to questioning and challenge. It enables midwives to consider different perspectives on issues.
- Because midwives are integral to the experience they are seeking to understand and part of the way in which they intervene in people's lives, they need to be able to think about how they impact on situations.
- The concern to develop ways of working that are women-centred and empowering – and the need for practice of and feedback on these – requires practitioners to be reflective.
- Reflective thinking sees as vital an exploration of feelings and their impact on one's approach. This sits well with midwifery, a profession where strong feelings about the task, the context and the people who use the services can be evoked.
- Reflective thinking can ensure that the linking of theory and practice is more than the technical applications of ideas – it also involves creative and flexible thinking.
- A reflective approach fits well with the complex nature of midwifery in which a range of perspectives needs to be incorporated.
- Adopting a reflective approach can be one way of keeping a focus on positive midwifery when faced with the pressures and constraints of practice.

- Reflective thinking can contribute to an understanding of the skills the midwife is using.
- Reflection can promote curiosity, which can lead to further learning.
(Duffy, 2007; Johns, 2009; Stuart, 2010; Taylor and White, 2000)

Reflection *in* action/reflection *on* action

Reflection may be used in practice in two main ways. Reflection *in* action involves thinking things through reflectively while also taking part in them. Examples might be reflection during a meeting with a woman, while supporting her birth experience, and while having a telephone conversation with her. This is a complex activity that we will explore more in Part Three. Reflection *on* action means thinking back on an event or an element piece of practice, as those mentioned previously, and thinking through what happened in a structured and systematic way. At this stage of the course it will be important to develop the habits of reflection *on* action – to routinely revisit experiences and explore them reflectively.

Case study: Linda learns about reflection on action

Sarah, Linda's current midwifery mentor, was asked to review a set of notes after a complaint had been made by a woman about a lack of communication during her birth experience. Linda had been present on that shift and thought she had good recall of the events as there had been a dramatic transfer to theatre in the second stage of labour resulting in a successful trial of instrumental labour. She had found the whole experience difficult, finding it hard to adapt to emergency theatre work as an inexperienced learner when really she wanted to be an efficient clinician able to respond rapidly to events and provide seamless care. Despite the advantage of previous experience of nursing adults, she was still uncomfortable being a student midwife during childbirth emergencies, particularly in theatre where her practice was observed by other hospital staff. She remembered her relief when the baby was born – crying loudly and in obvious good condition – without the need for a caesarean.

Linda recalled how busy her mentor Sarah had been during the theatre procedures, and how grateful the mother Karin and partner Chris had been immediately after the birth. She felt a little aggrieved for both her mentor and herself. Why were these people complaining now? She thought Sarah was more accepting of the complaint than she should be when they had both worked so hard during that birth.

Sarah went through the notes with Linda and then suggested that she reflect on the episode of care with particular focus on the experience for Karin and Chris and using the following questions.

- *What happened during the first and second stage of labour?*
- *What actions were carried out by me, as your mentor, and you, as a student? How did you communicate with both the couple and other team members? Were all interventions evidence-based and appropriate?*
- *What were your thoughts and feelings during the events surrounding the birth?*
- *Why did you think and feel this way?*
- *How might Karin and Chris have felt about the events and the communication with them?*
- *What were your thoughts afterwards?*
- *What theories and knowledge did you draw on?*
- *What values did you draw on?*

continued . . .

- *What have you learnt?*
- *What might you do differently next time?*

Sarah gave Linda some reading to help her to reflect on women's experience of care during difficult labours and births, and how these can impact on physical and psychological recovery after childbirth. Although Linda felt she was familiar with these issues, she was interested to read the literature on post-traumatic stress disorder relating to childbirth and learnt more about support services available to women and families.

When Linda had written her reflection on the episode for her log she realised that although, at the time, she had thought she had done her best, she had been preoccupied with her own performance and learning needs. Moreover, she had made assumptions about Karin's and Chris's awareness of the events to come and the safety of the baby.

Linda was aware of the current national policy drive to shift midwives from a clinical to a supportive role in theatres in the future (DH, 2010). For now she needed to work out a strategy that would help her cope with learning and responding to events in theatre while retaining the primary focus of working 'with woman'.

Students' experiences of being asked to be reflective

The benefits of becoming reflective thinkers are clear: students develop a deeper understanding of themselves and other factors, and how these insights impact on learning and practice. However, there is some evidence that suggests that students can find it a challenge.

- Thorpe (2000) found that some students were initially surprised that they were expected to be actively reflective and that tutors did not have all the answers.
- Stuart (2010) identified the difficulties midwifery students had in being reflective because of limited skills in 'noticing' both what was happening around them and within themselves. She commented: *Those who do not know how and what to notice may not be able to enter into the experience and will therefore be unable to enter into further reflective interaction with it* (p178). However, when students began to develop self-directed learning they became more skilled at analysing and reflecting.
- Stuart (2010) also observed during reflective workshops the distress experienced by midwifery students when recalling events that involved painful emotions evoked by interaction with people in life-and-death situations. She found, though, that the experience of sharing feelings enabled those feelings to be attended to more thoroughly. It then became possible to remove any obstructive ones and utilise those that were positive.
- Dearnley and Matthew (2007) found that some students had difficulty putting their thoughts in writing, but when they became more reflective they were able to connect with their prior knowledge and develop from a surface, procedural approach to a deeper level of understanding that included being able to challenge their existing ideas.

On your course you may be asked to participate in a number of learning activities designed to assist you to reflect – such as role play, simulation, reviewing videos of yourself, discussion and listening to different views, including those of people who use services. The evidence above suggests that although these might be initially uncomfortable and challenging, they are important in developing students' learning.

Activity 7.2   *Reflection*

Reflective learning

Think about how you have felt when asked to participate in activities in class that have been designed to help students to reflect. Try to list some reasons why you felt this way. Answering this honestly will involve you in some aspects of reflection. A reflective student will be developing self-awareness of why they respond to situations in particular ways.

Useful questions to promote reflection

When working towards becoming a reflective thinker it can be helpful to go about it in a systematic way, using questions to stimulate and promote your thinking.

Questions to help you think reflectively about a midwifery practice experience

Describe the experience

You could use these questions.

- What factors contributed to this experience occurring?
- What were significant background factors?
- What happened? What were the main components of the experience?
- What were your feelings, both positive and negative?
- What physical sensations were you aware of associated with these feelings?

Taking the time to do this gives you the opportunity to revisit what happened in a detailed way and become aware of issues you may have forgotten or set aside as not relevant. This is the *content* of the experience. To really engage in reflection you need to move on to thinking about the *process* of the experience.

Reflect on what happened during the experience

You could use the following questions.

- What was I trying to achieve?
- Why did I go about it in the way I did?
- What knowledge/theories did I bring to the situation?
- What values did I bring to the situation?

- How did my previous experiences affect what I thought and did? Did this situation remind me of similar ones?
- What were the consequences of my actions?
- How did I feel about the experience when it was happening?
- Why did I feel this way?
- What was the woman's perspective on the experience? How did she think and feel?
- How do I know that this was her perspective?
- Why was this her perspective?
- What was the perspective of others who were involved – for example, the woman's partner and family or other supporters?
- What factors influenced my decisions and actions during the experience?

Reflective thoughts after the experience

You could use the following questions.

- What was the impact of the way I went about this for the woman?
- What was the impact on me?
- What other choices did I have?
- What might have been the consequences of the other choices?

Learning from the experience

You could use the following questions.

- How do I feel now about the experience?
- Could I have dealt with it differently?
- What theories have I drawn on to help me understand this?
- What values have I drawn on to help me understand this?
- What gaps still exist in my understanding?
- What have I learnt from this that I might be able to use in new situations?
- What might get in the way of my doing things differently?

These questions add up to a long and comprehensive list, which demonstrates the depth and breadth that is important in reflective thinking. You may not always need to answer all the questions; however, when you first begin reflective thinking it is worth considering all of them.

You will find that reflective accounts of your practice experiences will be useful material for your placement portfolio and form part of your assessment, as they will provide evidence of your competence but also of your ability to think and analyse reflectively. You may also find that such accounts provide a helpful record of the development of your learning and could be included in your Personal Development Plan.

Case study: Linda supports Karin and Chris

This is a reflective account written by Linda using the questions above as a framework.

The experience

Sarah, my mentor, and I had taken over the care of Karin in established, spontaneous labour at 41+4 weeks of pregnancy. She was in the hospital delivery suite supported by her partner Chris and had laboured in the pool until her waters ruptured spontaneously and meconium was evident. To follow Trust Guidelines she got out of the pool to allow continuous monitoring. A few hours later when second stage was established by vaginal examination, thick meconium was present. A sudden marked bradycardia resulted in a rapid transfer to theatre for either an instrumental birth or a caesarean section. In theatre the fetal trace recovered, allowing a spinal anaesthetic to be sited, and an instrumental birth followed. The baby was born in good condition with satisfactory Apgar scores and cord gases. A week after the birth, Chris wrote a letter of complaint to the Head of Midwifery on behalf of Karin and himself.

Reflections on what happened

I was alarmed when the fetal heart rate dropped after the vaginal examination I carried out revealed that Karin was in the second stage of labour. When the heart rate did not recover despite maternal position change, my mentor rang the buzzer for help, and Karin was quickly transferred to theatre. I told Chris that we would come back for him with a gown and a hat, as supporters do not come into theatre until transfer is safely made and regional analgesia is successful. Immediately I felt out of place in theatre and was preoccupied with worrying that earlier I had missed something that might have alerted me to problems and avoided the dash to theatre. I helped Sarah with setting up theatre for an instrumental delivery, ensuring that the caesarean pack was ready – but I was anxious about remembering all the different pieces of equipment. I felt slightly nauseous and my hands were shaking. I watched my mentor carefully and tried to busy myself with the notes to calm my nerves – giving myself tasks. The anaesthetist and the obstetrician both asked me a question at the same time and I stumbled a bit in my reply and felt really stupid. I wanted to be back as a nurse in my nice, calm adult ward where I would be in full control!

The couple's experience

Now that I have read the complaint letter carefully, I can see that Karin felt abandoned in theatre. Although I was pleased she said some lovely things about the way we cared for her in the first stage of labour, I was then upset to read that she had felt we were more focused on preparing the theatre and writing notes than supporting her when she felt frightened and vulnerable. She said she simply hadn't understood what was happening. She could see that the staff were relieved and more relaxed when the fetal heart had recovered, but felt she wasn't given enough information or explanation and was quickly moved into a curled, left-lateral position for the spinal anaesthetic, which she found to be more painful and added to her sense of isolation. There was some loss of contact with the fetal heart at this point, and when the alarm on the cardiotocography consequently kept sounding she was really frightened that the baby might be very poorly or even die.

When Chris came to theatre she said he looked sick with worry – I didn't appreciate how alarmed he had been and assumed he would understand from our brief information and relaxed demeanour that the fetal heart had

continued . . .

improved. Although the staff looked cheery and some of them were chatting among themselves, I realise now that the couple were bewildered by this response and they thought it inappropriate. Karin also felt that she was exposed in front of a number of people in theatre who had not been introduced to her and whose roles she did not understand and that she was left in stirrups for a long time, with no cover over her, after the birth. Chris had felt isolated and extremely concerned about Karin when he was left alone in the pool room for a long time after the transfer to theatre. He could hear the screams of another woman and wasn't sure whether it was Karin. He said he had felt abandoned and was sure that something terrible was happening and that the baby might die.

Reflections on what happened

My aim had been, with Sarah, to support Karin and Chris during labour and birth, and ensure that both mother and baby were safe. I was trying to meet Karin's comfort needs and had given her lots of information about the physiology of birth, water birth and pain relief. I felt I had established a rapport with the couple and that Sarah trusted me to provide most of the care under her supervision. However, when the normal labour became more complex I began to feel out of my depth. When the transfer to theatre was inevitable I felt anxious about my role and my performance. I was really concerned for the couple and for the baby. But, on reflection, I realise that Sarah and I had not given enough information to the couple and that we had focused more on the practical considerations involved with the transfer. I had assumed that the couple would appreciate that we were trying to progress things and that they were in safe hands.

Learning from the experience

In future I will ensure that I discuss the implications of meconium more clearly with women and their families. Whenever a transfer to theatre is necessary I will give the woman and her supporters a realistic picture of events and a rough timeframe. As a student or qualified midwife I will ensure that the partner/relatives are kept informed (by me if possible) if there is a delay in theatre so they do not have additional worries about the safety of the woman and the baby during this separation.

I know I must accept that I am a learner and that I will become more fluid in emergencies and able to talk and perform at the same time. In the next theatre experience I will ensure that I do the basic tasks but also aim to spend more time reassuring the woman, being a positive presence, really trying to appreciate how she is interpreting events. I will endeavour to safeguard women's dignity wherever possible and with my mentor be ready to challenge other members of the team if their actions or presence are inappropriate. I will make every effort to spend time with women after the birth to go through what happened and maybe try to visit them the next day to talk things over.

On a practical level, after similar future events I will debrief with my mentor about what happened and discuss whether communication was effective. I will also produce some short checklists for myself as learning aids about procedures, equipment and theatre protocol.

I also need to be honest with myself and accept that in my past role as a nurse I was stressed and felt overwhelmed on occasions but was able to use my experience to deal with the inevitable uncertainties of dealing with people and changing health status – all part of the health carer's role.

Activity 7.3   *Reflection*

Practising reflection

Think back to a recent experience. It could be from your placement but it might be an experience in university. Practise thinking and writing reflectively by using the stages and questions set out above to record and explore the experience.

Tools to promote reflection

There are many ways you can develop as a reflective thinker, and on your course there will be activities and assessments focusing on reflection. Below are some ways of learning that you could use to develop your reflectiveness.

A reflective diary

Sometimes also called a reflective log or journal, this is different from a diary of events, which describes what happened. Rather, the writing in a reflective diary should be focused reflection on *selected* issues from your university or placement experience. These might be problems that are puzzling or troubling you, issues that fascinate you and you want to understand in greater depth, or experiences that you want to explore in greater depth – maybe because they went really well and you want to analyse why. Research by Collington and Hunt (2006) found that student midwives who kept reflective journals during their education programmes had adopted reflective practice in their working lives.

Case study: Nazneen's reflective diary

Nazneen had worked hard to avoid writing her diary in a descriptive way, aiming for a more reflective style, and was pleased to be getting good feedback from mentors and the midwifery course lecturers. She wanted to think more about a difficult episode of care that involved suturing advice when the woman had been challenging and unwilling to take advice. Nazneen thought that writing in her reflective diary about the events might be helpful.

Nazneen's reflective account

Together with my mentor Charlie I looked after Nina during her labour and birth at the end of her third pregnancy. The birth was straightforward but she sustained a labial tear that ended quite near the urethra and was initially bleeding quite profusely. However, Nina refused to have stitches, saying she had not needed them after her first two births; she was fed up with it all and didn't want any more 'horrible things when it should be all over' and she wanted to feed her baby. Nina was an older mother, articulate and well educated, and I felt quite intimidated by her assertiveness. I was also annoyed at the implication that the tear was somehow my fault as the birth attendant, because she had never had a tear before. I tried to point out that the blood loss was of concern and that the nature of the tear would mean that it could be quite painful for a few days, particularly whenever she passed urine. I found it difficult to get Nina to appreciate this and frustrating that she did not want to think

continued . . . •••

about possible future problems – she could only focus on avoiding the stitches now. I felt as if she was behaving like a teenager. Charlie, too, tried to talk Nina through the same information. In the time we spent talking to her the tear could have been easily repaired!

When Charlie looked again at the labial tear, the bleeding had settled down and Nina said triumphantly 'See!' as if everything was OK now. She continued to refuse to be sutured. We gave her lots of advice about hygiene, pain relief and signs of problems and said we would let the community midwife know about the issue.

Although I feel I was sensitive and appropriate with Nina, I now recognise that I was still feeling cross after we left her as I asked Charlie if I should get Nina to sign something to say that she took responsibility for her actions. Charlie was very kind and talked me through this response so I realised that I felt negative about Nina because she would not accept my advice. I also did actually feel guilty on some level that she had sustained a labial tear for the first time.

As it was a quiet shift I went through the following issues with Charlie.

- *The physiology of this particular birth and the reasons why an anterior tear might have occurred (an upright birth, which Nina had wanted to try for the first time, and a much larger baby than before).*
- *The healing process of perineal trauma and the actual risks that Nina would face (possibly minimal apart from comfort levels).*
- *Consent, choice and women's autonomy and an exploration of the concept of informed choice.*
- *Communication in difficult circumstances and when challenged.*
- *The importance of good record keeping and communication with the wider team.*

Charlie felt that Nina was, in fact, a very positive person and, rather than being critical of me, was expressing faith in her own body. She suggested that Nina was aware of her own particular way of coping even if things did not always work out as she anticipated. Charlie thought Nina was trying to plan for her own immediate needs and that she might be right in knowing what was best for her.

I can see that a blanket concept of 'informed choice' may be unrealistic in some circumstances and I need to think about the power relationship between the midwife and the woman and the weight given to the knowledge each holds. I had felt disempowered by Nina being so articulate and confident. Looking at it a different way, I can appreciate that women might feel the same in the face of an onslaught of advice from midwives or other professionals. It is rather unsettling to realise that, despite the best efforts of health carers to provide unbiased and evidence-based advice in a sensitive and appropriate way, women are also fully entitled to make uninformed choices, and we must work with this.

Reflective writing or discussion after watching video/DVD footage of yourself

Courses are increasingly using video cameras to assist students in the development of their communication and interpersonal skills. Once you have overcome the embarrassment of seeing yourself on the screen, it can be very helpful to take part in reflective discussion with other students and tutors about your skills. Another way of learning from seeing yourself on film is to write a reflective self-assessment afterwards.

Using a critical friend

Your own thinking and reflection can be sharpened if they are shared with someone else. The role of a critical friend is not to agree with you but to gently feed in suggestions about how the issue could be looked at from different angles.

Case study: Linda's critical friend

In Chapter 1 we noted how Linda had developed a critical friendship with Maggie, another student. This had been really helpful to both women. As the course progressed they continued to work together in this way. Their first placements were different – Maggie was working with a rural team in an affluent part of the county, with a high rate of normal births and home births, while Linda was placed in a busy city team where there were more women with higher obstetric risks and social problems.

In some ways this difference enabled them to avoid sympathising with each other; instead, they both kept a critical edge in their regular session.

Mentoring

During your practice learning your mentor should ensure that there is space for you to reflect on your placement experiences. A good mentor can really support the development of your reflective skills.

Tutorials

Small group or individual tutorials in university can provide you with a safe, supportive space in which to talk reflectively.

Taylor (2010) and Johns (2009) explore these tools and other ideas in more detail. Your course may advise you to use a particular model through which you can develop reflection – for example, Gibb's model, which is set out in Howatson-Jones (2013).

The qualities of reflective thinkers and practitioners

Activity 7.4   *Critical thinking*

The attributes of a reflective thinker

Make a list of what you consider to be the attributes of a reflective thinker.

Comment

The list of attributes of reflective thinkers below is put together from what writers on reflective thinking have suggested.

- Self-aware and with self-knowledge.
- Open to self-examination.
- Willing to take risks.
- Critically aware of how we have come to see the world in a particular way.
- Able to explain both how and why they have acted in a particular way.
- Able to take into account many different ways of looking at a situation.
- Able to synthesise – that is, to integrate new learning with what has been learnt before.
- Able to recognise and to manage emotions in themselves and others – emotional intelligence.
- Curious about the impact of themselves.
- Motivated to develop and improve practice.
- Prepared to devote time to reflection.
- Able to think in a holistic, integrated and multi-layered way and so respond sensitively to unique and unpredictable situations in midwifery practice.
  (Boud et al.,1985; Moon, 2004; Stuart, 2010; Thorpe, 2000)

Activity 7.5   *Decision making*

Developing as a reflective learner

Using the list above, identify the ways in which you could develop to become a more reflective learner.

Writing reflectively

In addition to thinking reflectively, you will, during your course, be required to write reflectively. As discussed earlier, reflective writing will be expected as part of your evidence in your practice portfolio. You might also, within an essay or assignment, be asked to reflect on your own skills, your use of theories and approaches, and your responses to service users, colleagues and other professionals. Reflective writing may be included in your Personal Development Plan (Bolton, 2010).

Reflective writing demands a different writing style from other types of academic writing as it:

- builds on descriptive writing;
- uses theory and knowledge but goes beyond this;
- is exploratory;
- asks questions but does not always have the answers;
- incorporates emotional content – explores feelings;
- brings in values – both personal and professional;

- considers different ways of looking at a situation;
- involves thinking deeply;
- demands you challenge yourself;
- can be uncomfortable.

Because reflective writing is an account of your journey of reflection it is acceptable to write in the first person – that is, using 'I'.

Students sometimes find reflective writing challenging for the following reasons.

- Having learnt how to write academically, they are then expected to write in another way.
- It is exploratory and can involve revealing aspects of yourself you might feel reticent about sharing – such as doubts, prejudices and strong feelings.
- It involves writing in the first person, which some people find uncomfortable and unfamiliar. Some women students have said that they simply find it difficult to put themselves first.

Some pitfalls in reflective writing

- In reflective writing students are encouraged to explore their feelings, values and assumptions, so there can be a tendency for the assignment to include material about themselves without making any connections to theories, concepts, principles or values. The tutor reading this is likely to see it as self-indulgent exploration rather than true reflective writing. You can avoid this by always connecting your reflections to established frameworks for thinking.
- Sometimes students end a piece of writing with the phrase *my reflections on this are* and then continue with writing that does not show any of the characteristics of reflection. For example: *My reflections after the event were that this interview went well and Mrs Jones went away happy.* Hopefully you can see that while this includes the word *reflections* it does not meet the basic criteria for reflective writing.
- The reflective writing takes up a disproportionate amount of the assignment. It is essential that you study with care the essay or assignment guidelines and assessment criteria so you are clear about what you are expected to achieve in the submitted piece of work.
- It can be easy to make unrealistic statements about your future learning and practice – for example, *in future I will always give women my full support when they don't follow my advice.* Make sure you make realistic statements and acknowledge the complexity of your current and future practice.
- Reflection occurs at the end of an assignment rather than being integrated throughout the written work. A truly reflective piece of work will interweave theory, practice, values and reflection – all appropriately referenced.

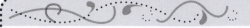

Chapter summary

In this chapter we have explored reflective thinking and its importance in both learning about and practising midwifery. Our focus has been on reflection on action – reflecting after the event. It has become clear that important features of reflection are, first, the incorporation of feelings and, second, how learning can emerge from reflection. Some of the challenges of reflection have been explored, including the different style of writing that will be needed. A series of questions that you can use to assist you in the reflective process has been provided, together with some examples. Reflection is a key skill for midwives. However, on its own it is not sufficient: reflection needs to be blended with knowledge, theory, values, practice skills and research. In Part Three we will give more consideration to reflection, particularly reflection in action and synthesising reflection with other forms of knowledge.

Further reading

Bolton, G (2010) *Reflective practice: writing and professional development*. London: Sage.

This book focuses particularly on using reflective writing to promote understanding and learning. It includes some helpful ideas and activities for developing reflective writing.

Howatson-Jones, L (2013) *Reflective practice in nursing* (2nd edition). Exeter: Learning Matters.

Jasper, M (2013) *Beginning reflective practice* (2nd edition). Andover: Cengage.

Johns, C (2009) *Becoming a reflective practitioner*. Oxford: Wiley Blackwell.

Taylor, B (**2010**) *Reflective practice for healthcare professionals*. Maidenhead: McGraw Hill.

These four titles all give good introductions to the subject.

Chapter 8
Understanding and using research

This chapter will help you to meet the Quality Assurance Agency for Higher Education (2008) requirement that students studying at Level 5 are able to:

- demonstrate knowledge of the main methods of enquiry in the subject(s) relevant to the named award, and ability to evaluate critically the appropriateness of different approaches to solving problems in the field of study;
- effectively communicate information, arguments and analysis in a variety of forms to specialist and non-specialist audiences and deploy key techniques of the discipline effectively.

NMC Standards for Pre-registration Midwifery Education

This chapter will address the following competencies:

Domain: Effective midwifery practice

Determine and provide programmes of care and support for women which:

- are based on best evidence and clinical judgment.

Provide seamless care and, where appropriate, interventions, in partnership with women and other care providers during the antenatal period which:

- are evidence based.

These will include:

- ensuring that current research findings and other evidence are incorporated into practice.

Work in partnership with women and other care providers during the postnatal period to provide seamless care and interventions which:

- are evidence based.

continued . . .

Contribute to enhancing the health and social wellbeing of individuals and their communities. This will include:

- informing practice using the best evidence which is shown to prevent and reduce maternal and perinatal morbidity and mortality.

Domain: Achieving quality care through evaluation and research

Inform and develop the midwife's own practice and the practice of others through using the best available evidence and reflecting on practice. This will include:

- keeping up to date with evidence;
- applying evidence to practice.

Chapter aims

After reading this chapter you will be able to:

- appreciate what is meant by research in academic study;
- understand the contribution of research to developing knowledge and practice in midwifery;
- be aware of debates about the role of research in midwifery.

Introduction

Midwives draw on different types of knowledge to inform their practice. Cluett and Bluff (2006) categorise them in these ways.

- *Traditional knowledge*, which is passed on from midwife to midwife through generations and is based on the values and beliefs of midwifery. It includes the 'ways things are done' in the hospital and the policies associated with the medical model of care.
- *Knowledge derived from clinical experience*, which derives from experience but also, as we have noted in Chapter 7, from thoughtful reflection on that experience.
- *Personal knowledge*, which is knowing one's self, thus contributing to midwifery practice that is more authentic and self-aware about our impact on others – colleagues and the women and families we work with.
- *Intuitive knowledge*, which is sometimes referred to as gut-feeling. A better term might be tacit knowledge – what we have learnt but is not readily articulated. Reflection and critical thinking can uncover the basis of this knowledge.
- *Empirical knowledge*, which is what Eraut calls propositional knowledge (see Chapter 6, page 81). It is generated through research and is used to guide practice.

We suggest that other important types of knowledge for midwifery practice include the following.

- *Knowledge from women and their families*, which is what midwives can learn from people who have used their services.
- *Organisational knowledge*, which is about the governance and regulation frameworks that shape midwifery practice.
- *Policy knowledge*, which is about how midwifery fits into the complex social, political and economic environment.

All these types of knowledge, in different ways, can contribute to evidence-based practice in midwifery. In earlier chapters we have considered theories, statistics, knowledge derived from midwives and the experiences of people using midwifery services, together with knowledge generated through reflection. In this chapter we will focus on knowledge developed through research. Although research has been mentioned in earlier chapters, we have not explored in detail what is understood by it in academic study. In this chapter we will begin to consider the role of research in developing knowledge and guiding practice in midwifery. At the next stage of the degree you need to be able to use, comment on and critically evaluate research. The topic of research in this chapter is therefore continued in the next part of the book.

Research can be a daunting topic to study, partly because of the technical language used. We have aimed to set out this out in a clear and accessible way. However, you may also find it helpful to refer to other texts that explore midwifery and nursing research; some examples can be found at the end of the chapter. Of these, you might find that Tracey Ross's (2012) book is the most useful, particularly the 'jargon-busting' sections at the end of each of her chapters.

What is research?

A general definition of research is provided by the *Concise Oxford Dictionary* (11th edition) (2008):

> *The systematic investigation into and study of material sources etc in order to establish facts and reach new conclusions.*

So the key aspects of research are that its purposes are to find things out and create new knowledge, and that the way that this is done should be organised and structured. This may entail using existing information. Cluett and Bluff (2006, p20) note the importance of the relationship of research to practice:

> *research is a process that strives to increase and validate knowledge, thus contributing to the provision of evidence on which to base midwifery theories and practice.*

Meanwhile, Downe (2012, p7) asserts:

> *The whole aim of our research endeavour is to provide the evidence to maximise positive childbirth for women, babies, families and maternity care staff.*

Finding new things out through midwifery research is therefore clearly linked to the desire to influence and improve practice.

Activity 8.1   *Reflection*

Midwifery research

Make a list of:

- what you think the purposes of research might be;
- issues that research in midwifery might explore.

Comment

Cluett and Bluff (2006) suggest the purposes of research are:

- to deepen understanding of the physiological, psychological and sociological aspects of child-bearing;
- to develop a sound and reasoned foundation for midwifery practice;
- to increase the choices for women and their families;
- to develop standards of care and contribute to the quality of services;
- to contribute to the cost-effectiveness of care.

A historical note

Midwifery and midwifery knowledge have 'ancient' traditions (Cluett and Bluff, 2006), and specific research in midwifery has been relatively recent in comparison with its history. Practitioner knowledge and research from medicine were previously its foundations. In the last 40 years these foundations have been expanded. The 1972 Briggs Report (DHSS, 1972) stated that all health-related care should be research based, although at this time the focus of midwifery research tended to be the role of the midwife and the numbers needed to provide care. In the mid to late 1970s midwives themselves began to undertake research, and this development widened the scope of the purpose and topics of research. Developments such as the National Midwifery Database and the Cochrane pregnancy and childbirth database have strengthened the quality and quantity of research. These changes were part of the growth of an evidence-based practice emphasis in all health care. However, there was a risk of 'evidence' being seen as the same thing as research, with only some types of research (particularly randomised controlled trials) being seen as valid approaches. Despite this, a broad view is now taken of what can be valid evidence, and midwifery research has flourished in its quality, range and diversity – now covering all aspects of midwifery practice.

Issues midwifery research might explore

Different groups of people

- Women.
- Families.
- Babies.
- Midwives.
- Other members of the obstetric team.

Developing understanding of particular issues and experiences

- Aspects of pregnancy and childbirth.
- Aspects of practice: what might promote safer births and reduce mortality.
- The experience of women when using services.
- The experiences of families.
- The experiences of midwives in different contexts.
- Ethical aspects of practice.
- What might be of benefit to women in childbearing, physically and psychologically.
- How public health initiatives might be promoted.
- Teaching and learning in midwifery.

It is clear that midwifery research is broad in its range, creating new insights into many topics and issues that you might find useful in your degree studies.

Activity 8.2 *Reflection*

How research might be useful

Think of an issue you have come across on your placement about which you would have welcomed some research in order to help you understand it better.

Case study: Paul and the third stage of labour

Paul found the third stage of labour fascinating. He had observed huge variations in women's expectations and responses to this important part of the birth: some were very engaged and interested while others appeared to barely notice it. In addition, he had seen midwifery mentors and medical staff using different techniques. In order to develop his understanding he looked at the research on the third stage. This developed his grasp of the complexity of the topic – for example, about what was the best intervention in the third stage in terms of reducing blood loss (Begley et al., 2011). Of particular interest was the material on the effects of early cord clamping on neonatal outcomes and subsequent discussions with mentors about how some practitioners changed the way they dealt with the third stage as a result of the growing research evidence (Andersson et al., 2011).

Approaches to research or methodologies

Research methodology is concerned with the theoretical and philosophical assumptions that can be made about the knowledge that is produced from the research (Steen and Roberts, 2011). It is usually subdivided into qualitative and quantitative research, and we will consider each in turn. Some research projects combine both methodologies. Research methods – which will be discussed later – are the different ways in which the data for analysis is collected. Not all research texts make a distinction between methodology and methods, but understanding the difference is important and can be helpful when critically evaluating research.

Activity 8.3   *Critical thinking*

Research methodology

Find the most recent edition of a journal such as *Midwifery, Evidence Based Midwifery* or *British Journal of Midwifery.* Select an article that is an account of a piece of midwifery research and of interest to you. Read it through. Then read the next section of this chapter. When you have finished, try to identify the approaches to research or methodologies used.

Qualitative research

Qualitative research tends to focus on experiences, thoughts and behaviour from the perspective of the participants. It focuses on the meaning of events, interventions and issues for those being researched. It does not aim for disinterested objectivity, and it recognises the subjective position of the researcher in the research project. Walsh (2007) asserts that the value of qualitative research is in its power to explain complex phenomena and provide a new way of seeing things that can help to enhance practice.

Ethnographic research

The intention of ethnographic research is to understand people's behaviour in their context and culture. Data is collected by researchers who immerse themselves in, and observe, a situation in order to understand it more fully. It is an attempt to capture the subtleties behind formal and official accounts of organisations or institutions and to reveal what is often not documented. Because it is very difficult to be in a situation and not influence it, researchers need to be self-aware of what they bring to the observation. Examples would be studies of how midwives practise in relation to particular groups of people or aspects of pregnancy and childbirth.

Example: Newburn, M (2012) The best of both worlds: parents' motivations for using an alongside birth centre from an ethnographic study. *Midwifery*, 28 (1): 61–66

The researchers in this study spent many hours at a birth centre observing care and carrying out in-depth interviews with women and families and staff. When Paul – one of the three midwifery students we are following – read this article he concluded that the approach taken to the research had been important in generating the findings and this added to the large body of literature already emphasising the importance of a calm, nurturing and home-like atmosphere for women in labour. The findings certainly corresponded to his reflections during a placement in an alongside midwifery-led unit.

Phenomenological research

Phenomenological research aims to describe how people see a particular situation or experience from their perspective. The researcher aims to put aside their own preconceived thoughts or knowledge – many research studies explicitly discuss this process so it is open for criticism and debate.

Example: Nyman,V, Downe, S and Berg, M (2011) Waiting for permission to enter the labour ward world: first-time parents' experiences of the first encounter on a labour ward. *Sexual & Reproductive Healthcare*, 2: 129–34

The aim of this Swedish study was to explore the meaning of the first encounter of first-time mothers and their partners with midwives and other maternity care staff when they arrived on a hospital labour ward. The researchers acknowledged that they started from the perspective that the first encounter is a highly significant moment for the midwife and the couple that has the potential to turn their anxiety and uncertainty about the coming labour into confidence and hope, or to reinforce fear and anxiety. The data was collected via interviews and focus groups, which, it was felt, were helpful ways of capturing the meanings of the first encounter for the women and their partners. The study concluded that this first encounter was typified by waiting for permission to enter and to stay on the labour ward, in response to rules that the women and their partners did not necessarily understand, and which did not seem to take account of their specific worries, concerns and support needs.

Another of our midwifery students, Linda, had found this study in a search for background reading for her placement in the triage unit at the main maternity hospital. She found the researchers' approach was really revealing about what the experience of the labour ward could be for women and their families – something that could easily be missed in busy shifts. Some of the behaviours of women and staff described by the authors were immediately recognisable. Institutionalised systems to assess need and offer help seemed to create issues of power and control. Sometimes women responded by behaving in ways they thought caregivers would see as appropriate. Linda began to think of ways that she could use this additional knowledge to improve initial encounters with clients and information sharing with them.

Grounded theory

Grounded theory aims to develop theory about a particular issue by studying people's perceptions or interactions and by systematically analysing the data. It starts without preconceived ideas and builds theory from the data collected.

Example: Lipp, A (2010) Conceding and concealing judgement in termination of pregnancy; a grounded theory study. *Journal of Research in Nursing*, 15 (4): 365–78

This research aimed to explore nurses' feelings when working with the termination of pregnancy. Grounded theory was chosen because it enabled a systematic analysis and development of theory from a mass of data gathered through interviews on a topic that is relatively unexplored. As the interviews progressed, themes that had theoretical relevance emerged. These were: conceding judgement; concealing judgement; the different approaches to repeat terminations; and the use of maxims to conceal judgement.

Before reading the research Nazneen had done much soul searching about her own attitudes and feelings after being involved in a termination on her placement. She could see how using a grounded theory approach had developed an understanding of midwives' views by identifying broad themes on this complex issue.

Case study research

Case study research takes one particular issue, situation or phenomena and explores it in depth and detail in order to understand it better. Examples might be one birth experience, one booking-in appointment and one midwifery-led unit.

Example: Dow, A (2012) Simulation-based learning: a case study, part 3. *British Journal of Midwifery*, 20 (9): 654–58

This research aimed to explore the role of clinical simulation in one specific situation involving a university skills laboratory designed to reflect the local maternity unit's labour and delivery room. A small sample of midwifery lecturers (2), students (6) and mentors (7) were interviewed. In this article, the third of three, the impact of clinical simulation on learning in the workplace is discussed. The conclusions reached were that learning through simulation in the university was positively evaluated by all those interviewed; it was helpful when student midwives began to learn in a clinical environment and made the interface between university and practice placement more manageable. The article notes the drawbacks of reaching conclusions from one small case study because the findings may be limited to this particular study site.

Quantitative research

Quantitative research, in contrast to qualitative research, is concerned with what can be measured objectively: facts, figures and experiments. It often sets out to test a hypothesis and so takes a deductive approach to the development of knowledge. It is used when facts and figures might be helpful to resolve a situation or determine the best approach.

Randomised controlled trials (RCTs)

This methodology has been used extensively in medical research and has been seen as the 'gold standard' in producing the most reliable scientific evidence. In RCTs two groups are compared in order to test the effectiveness of an intervention. They focus on factors that are measurable.

Participants in the trial are selected and allocated to each group randomly in order that other factors that might impact on the findings are evenly distributed. Ideally, participants, clinicians and researchers should be unaware of which intervention 'arm' of the trial the participant has been allocated to ('double blinding') until the trial is over, but this is not always possible. Even if participants drop out of the study or use another intervention, their outcomes are often analysed with the rest of the group that they were originally allocated to – this is called 'intention to treat'. The mathematic analysis of the difference in outcomes of the intervention groups has more validity if the numbers in each group are very large. Well-designed large RCTs should reduce bias and eliminate the possibility of an associated factor blurring the results. They can, however, be costly and time-consuming, and some subjects cannot be considered because of ethical problems or the problem of 'blinding' participants. In pregnancy and childbirth, women often have clear views about participating in research, or about the type of intervention they want to choose, and this may skew the validity of results.

Example: Hannah, M E, Hannah, W J, Hewson, S, Hodnett, E, Saigal, S, Willan, A for the Term Breech Trial Collaborative Group (2000) Planned caesarean section versus planned vaginal birth for breech presentation at term: a randomised multicentre trial. *Lancet* (356) 1375–83

The researchers aimed to compare the outcomes for women having planned caesarean sections and those having planned vaginal birth when the baby is presenting as breech, and 2,088 women in 121 centres across 26 countries were randomly allocated to either a caesarean section or a vaginal birth. They were followed up six weeks after birth. The findings were that, for the baby, perinatal mortality, neonatal mortality and serious neonatal morbidity were lower in the group delivered by planned section. For the women there was no significant difference in maternal mortality or serious maternal morbidity.

Nazneen was aware of the powerful effect that this trial had had on the way in which breech presentation is managed in the UK and across the world. The trial involved very large numbers, which increased the validity, and it was an international, multi-centred project published in a high-status journal. Her link lecturer drew her attention to literature that responded to the Term Breech Trial, some of which criticised the methodology and raised questions about its validity for clinical decision making. There seemed to be growing concerns about short- and long-term maternal morbidity as a result of the increase in caesarean sections for breech presentations as an outcome of the trial.

Nazneen spent some time in placement at the local Trust's external cephalic version (ECV) clinic and observed discussions with women about the risks of breech birth and how the evidence from the trial was used.

Cohort studies

These are studies of people over a long period of time to identify changes. Comparison is made with another group that does not have the condition or did not receive the treatment or intervention. The issue being considered must be measurable.

Example: Brocklehurst, P et al. (Birthplace in England Collaborative Group) (2011) Perinatal and maternal outcomes by planned place of birth for healthy women with low risk pregnancies: the Birthplace in England national prospective cohort study. *British Medical Journal*, 343: d7400: 1–13

This study followed a large cohort of women (57,000) who were healthy and had low-risk pregnancies from the start of care in pregnancy through to after birth. Linda had been on placement at a freestanding midwifery-led unit (MLU) when the Birthplace Study results were published. She could see the value of research that tracked women in this way and was impressed by the size of the cohort, which strengthened the validity of the findings. The midwives Linda was working with were very interested in the results and pleased to see that birth at home and in MLUs had been shown to be safe for low-risk women. The study did show that perinatal outcomes were poorer for first-time mothers, and there was lively debate in the unit about the evidence for this. The findings on the impact of transfer in labour for women prompted Linda to discuss strategies with her mentor on decision making for transfer and planning communication with women and families in these circumstances.

Data collection or methods in research

Activity 8.4   *Critical thinking*

Research methods

List the ways or methods you think might be used to collect data in midwifery research. Then read the next section of the chapter. When you have finished, check your list against the methods outlined here.

'Research methods' is the term used to describe the range of ways in which data or information for a research study is collected. The methods that are chosen when the researchers plan their studies should be related to the research methodology. They should provide the best way of gathering the kind of data that will throw light on the topic the researchers are investigating.

Interviews

Interviews are face-to-face encounters between a researcher/interviewer and a respondent, and are most often used in qualitative research. Some interviewers, particularly those carrying out surveys, will use a standardised questionnaire, while others will adopt a less fixed approach. This might entail a semi-structured interview based on a small number of open-ended questions; the researcher may ask for elaboration by asking more specific questions. In unstructured interviews the interviewer allows the interviewee free range to give an account in their own way, although the interviewer may probe for more depth and detail and seek clarification. Interviews are normally recorded. Feminist researchers have asserted that interviews are unlikely to be objective, arguing that the personal characteristics of the interviewer and respondent, and a degree of closeness between them, are important to the interview process. However, interviews can produce rich data about people's experiences and feelings.

Example: McCutcheon, R and Brown, D (2012) A qualitative exploration of women's experiences of giving birth at home. *Evidence Based Midwifery*, 10 (1): 23–28

These researchers wanted to develop knowledge of women's experiences of giving birth at home. In order to gather their information they carried out in-depth semi-structured interviews using open-ended questions with nine women. Private spaces chosen by the women were used for the interviews, which were audio-taped to enable analysis of the data generated using a grounded theory methodology. The theory this developed suggested that women adopt a philosophy of control in planning and giving birth at home. This includes three stages: preparing for the challenges, developing resilience strategies and reviewing the outcome of the home birth experience.

Focus groups

Focus groups are a useful and effective way of ascertaining views from a group of people together. The researcher puts issues and questions to the group, which will explore them and present their views. As the focus group progresses, perspectives can change through the process of exchange of views and discussion, and researchers need to be aware of this, and record and analyse this along with other data produced. Virtual online focus groups can also be used for research.

Example: Kerrigan, A and Houghton, G (2010) Including marginalised groups in maternity research: the challenges for midwives. *Evidence Based Midwifery*, 8 (1): 4–7

This research was carried out in order to improve women's access to information during pregnancy in a diverse, multicultural area where many women were not aware of all the services available to them. In order to ensure as wide participation as possible, the researcher worked through children's centres, a community worker and clinics, including a 'link clinic' for women whose first language is not English, to set up focus groups. The discussion in the focus groups generated data from a wide range of women.

Observation

Researchers may collect data by observing an activity or practice. Qualitative data is generally produced by open-ended observation. Observation that is more structured and defined can be used to generate quantitative data – for example, how often an event occurs during a pre-determined time. Participant observation occurs when a researcher is part of the event or activity they are observing. This can be helpful because the context and the culture can be appreciated by the 'insider' researcher. There is, however, a risk of the researcher being over-subjective and not sufficiently aware or reflective about this.

Example: Radcliffe, P (2011) Substance-misusing women: stigma in the maternity setting. *British Journal of Midwifery*, **19 (8): 497–506**

The aim of this research was to explore the workplace discourse of antenatal staff in caring for substance-misusing women. The data was gathered through interviews but also through non-participative observation of clinical settings and staff meetings. The researcher observed the following: three afternoon sessions of a hospital-based clinic for opiate-using pregnant women; three multidisciplinary meetings at which midwives, postnatal ward sisters, care managers and drug and alcohol workers discussed their caseload of substance-misusing patients; a community midwife's caseload on one day, which included home visits and antenatal appointments of twelve non-substance misusing women and five antenatal midwifery appointments and scans with substance-misusing women. The researcher found that workplace discourse in antenatal services may reinforce views of substance-misusing or methadone-prescribed women as unreliable and risky. However, midwives and antenatal professionals who had developed specialist knowledge or who had received training on the social and emotional experience of substance-misusing/methadone-prescribed women were more accepting and empathetic and less likely to resort to stereotypes.

Questionnaires

Questionnaires can be a structured way of gathering either quantitative or qualitative information. They may be used in face-to-face interviews, as discussed above, or sent out by post. They are a good means of systematically gathering information from a large number of people. Data gained from questionnaires may be both qualitative and quantitative. The design of the questionnaire should be dependent on the aims and approach of the research.

Example of quantitative data from questionnaires: McCowan, L M E, Dekker, G A, Chan, E, Stewart, A, Chappell, L C, Hunter, M, Moss-Morris, R and North, R A (2009) Spontaneous preterm birth and small for gestational age infants in women who stop smoking early in pregnancy: prospective cohort study. *British Medical Journal*, **338: b1081**

The objective of this study was to compare pregnancy outcomes of women who stopped smoking in early pregnancy and those who either did not smoke in pregnancy or who continued to smoke. A research midwife, using a questionnaire, interviewed all the women who were recruited into the trial at 15 weeks and then at 20 weeks. The women also completed a lifestyle questionnaire that used psychological scales to measure anxiety and depression. Data from the 15 weeks' interviews was entered into a database, and participants were followed up prospectively, with pregnancy outcome data and baby measurements collected by research midwives, usually within 72 hours of birth.

Analysis of the data showed that women who stopped smoking before 15 weeks' gestation had rates of spontaneous pre-term birth and small-for-gestational-age infants that did not differ from those of non-smokers. The rates for women who continued to smoke were significantly higher. The study concluded that adverse effects of smoking may be reversible if smoking is stopped early in pregnancy. A criticism of a questionnaire could be the reliability on the accuracy of self-reporting. This is particularly important in sensitive areas such as smoking in pregnancy, where women may fear judgement from the interviewer regarding her responses. Although the study did not measure cotinine levels, the researchers state that the very similar outcomes for both stopped smokers and non-smokers validate the claims of women who said they had stopped smoking.

Example of qualitative data from questionnaires: Baxter, J and Pride, J (2008) Should midwives wear uniforms? Let's ask the women. *British Journal of Midwifery*, **16 (8): 523–26**

The purpose of this study was to obtain the views of women about whether midwives at a London hospital should wear uniforms when midwives had a choice between their own clothes, nurse-type uniforms and theatre blues. Questionnaires were given to 115 women leaving the hospital and a high response rate (91 per cent) was achieved. Views were divided evenly. Key themes identified in the responses were professional identity, safety and caring being more important than uniforms.

Action research

Action research is a kind of applied research. It is focused on bringing about change in a policy or practice and is research on actions taken. Often the researcher may be implementing the change as well as studying its effect or impact. It aims to produce practical knowledge and does not claim to be objective or free of bias.

Example: Madden, E, Sinclair, M and Wright, M (2011) Teamwork in obstetric emergencies. *Evidence Based Midwifery*, **9 (3): 95–101**

This study set out to find out more about how to increase the effectiveness and efficiency of team-working when obstetric emergencies occur. To achieve this, obstetric emergencies were simulated and video-recorded to explore the interaction, behaviour and practices of healthcare professionals within a framework of peer support. Data from the video clips were examined, and emerging themes were identified and agreed. As a result, changes were agreed and made to practice and procedures around communication, collaboration and control that improved responses to obstetric emergencies.

Using existing documents and data

This method uses data that already exists in the forms of statistics and documents (sometimes historical) to find out more about a topic. Examples of documents that might be considered in midwifery research are current or historical midwifery textbooks, policy documents, hospital/ medical records and midwifery journals. The information gleaned from these documents is then used in exploring answers to the research question. Sometimes the researcher will ask people to keep diaries on a particular issue, and these documents are used as the data for the research.

Example of data collection: Office for National Statistics (2013) *Statistical bulletin: Live births in England and Wales by characteristics of mother 1. 2011.* **London: The Stationery Office**

Data from birth registrations in England and Wales in 2011 by characteristics of the mother is presented in this statistical bulletin. Key findings included the following.

- In 2011, nearly half (49 per cent) of all live births were to mothers aged 30 and over.
- Nearly two-thirds (65 per cent) of fathers were aged 30 and over in 2011 (excluding births registered solely by the mother).
- In 2011, 84 per cent of babies were registered by parents who were married, in a civil partnership or cohabiting.
- In 2011, the standardised average (mean) age of mothers for all births was 29.7 years.
- For first births the standardised average (mean) age of mothers was 27.9 years.

Example of using diaries in research: Way, S (2011) The combined use of diaries and interviewing for the collection of data in midwifery research. *Evidence Based Midwifery,* **9 (2): 66–70**

In this research diaries were used in addition to interviews to explore women's experience of perineal trauma. Women were asked to keep a diary for ten days following the birth of their baby and describe what effect this had on being able to carry out daily living activities such as walking, sitting and feeding their baby. Diaries were chosen as a method for collecting data as they provided the opportunity for the women to write about their thoughts and feelings as close to their experience as possible. To obtain greater depth, detail and clarity, the same women were then invited to explore through interview the experiences they had described. Women in the study appeared to welcome the opportunity to write about their birth experience and additionally used it to reflect on their journey of recovery during the early postnatal period.

Reviews and metasyntheses

Research reviews locate, evaluate, explore and summarise all the known research on a particular topic in order to identify the best possible guide to practice. They tend to use quantitative research. The Cochrane Library is a major source of reviews.

Example: Jones, L, Othman, M, Dowswell, T, Alfirevic, Z, Gates, S, Newburn, M, Jordan, S, Lavender, T and Neilson, J P (2012) Pain management for women in labour: an overview of systematic reviews. *Cochrane Database of Systematic Reviews* **Issue 3. Art. No. CD009234. DOI: 10.1002/14651858.CD009234.pub2**

This review of research into pain management in labour searched sources to identify all relevant systematic reviews of randomised controlled trials. It identified 15 Cochrane reviews (255 included trials) and three non-Cochrane reviews (55 included trials) for inclusion within the overview.

When he read the review findings, Paul was not surprised to discover the limited research carried out on non-pharmacological forms of pain relief or comfort in labour. He noted, however, some evidence for the benefits of immersion in water, acupuncture and massage. He was interested to see that there was insufficient evidence to make a judgement on whether TENS was effective for pain relief in labour.

Metasyntheses undertake in-depth analysis of a number of research studies on related topics in order to integrate the findings and draw conclusions.

Example: O'Connell, R and Downe, S (2009) A metasynthesis of midwives' experience of hospital practice in publicly funded settings: compliance, resistance and authenticity. *Health*, 13 (6): 589–609

O'Connell and Downe wanted to explore what research revealed about how midwives perceived hospital midwifery, particularly focusing on practice in labour wards, and to find out the narratives they used to explain their work. Fourteen studies were selected, and three overarching themes were identified from the analysis of them: 'power and control'; 'compliance with cultural norms'; and 'attempting to normalise birth'. While most midwives aimed to provide what they called 'real midwifery', this intention was often overwhelmed by heavy workloads and the pressure to provide equitable care to all women. Linda found it fascinating that these findings emerged from a **synthesis** of many studies. The themes were familiar to her from her own reading and practice experience on the triage unit at her local hospital. Linda wondered about the value of research if the findings were not noted or acted upon by funders and policy makers.

Useful sources of research for midwifery students

In order to be able to use relevant research it is helpful to be aware of useful sources. Because a good deal of research is written in a style suitable for academic journals rather than being focused on helping students to learn, it can be difficult initially to begin to find your way into using research. Your degree course will contain a strong research element and tutors will provide direction. University librarians will also guide and support you in accessing databases and electronic journals.

Activity 8.5   *Research and finding out*

Using other people's studies

List the sources of midwifery research material that you have used on placement or for your assignments. Then check against the sources identified below.

Research summaries: One way of beginning is to become familiar with the range of research available and its potential usefulness by drawing on summaries. These can be found in: *British Journal of Midwifery, MIDIRS* and *Essentially MIDIRS*, and medical journals such as *British Medical Journal* and *The Lancet*.

Midwifery journals: Journals that contain fuller accounts of research in article form are: *The Practising Midwife; MIDIRS* and *Essentially MIDIRS; Evidence Based Midwifery*; and *British Journal of Midwifery*.

Websites: Current and recent articles in the above journals can be found online using access provided through university libraries or individual subscriptions. In addition, useful websites include the following.

- *The Cochrane Library* is a collection of databases of high-quality, independent evidence to inform healthcare decision making. The databases contain systematic reviews on many aspects of healthcare, including those produced by the Pregnancy and Childbirth Group, which analyses all good quality studies and their results on each issue and assesses whether meaningful conclusions can be drawn. There is a plain English summary for every review, but the discussion on the methodology and validity of each piece of research is usually very accessible. Go to: http://onlinelibrary.wiley.com/o/cochrane/clabout/articles/PREG/frame.html.
- *NICE (The National Institute for Health and Care Excellence)* develops guidance on an enormous range of health topics, including many maternity-specific issues such as antenatal care, pregnancy and birth and postnatal care. NICE develops recommendations on topics chosen by the Department of Health using the best available evidence, which includes the views of experts, patients and carers, and industry. The guidance is then created by independent and unbiased advisory committees. Go to: www.nice.org.uk/.
- *NHS Choices: Behind the headlines* is a very useful service that gives an unbiased and evidence-based analysis of many of the health stories that make the news. In clear, accessible language, the NHS Choices Teams provide a really useful description of the research methodology that was used in the original research and how the team weighs the evidence to assess whether the results and the consequent media conclusions are valid. At the start of 2013, the team had covered more than 500 stories on pregnancy/child issues. Go to: www.nhs.uk/news/Pages/NewsIndex.aspx.
- Sites such as studentmidwife.net can offer support and dialogue between students on research and assignments in a relaxed and non-threatening way.

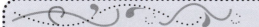

Chapter summary

This chapter has been an introduction to the knowledge for evidence-based practice that is generated through research. It has explored briefly different methodologies and methods of research providing examples as illustrations. However, other aspects of research also require consideration, in particular the ethics of research. In the next chapter we will again consider research and how to evaluate it for use in midwifery practice.

Further reading

Most standard midwifery textbooks will contain a chapter providing a basic outline on research or evidence-based practice. All of the following provide a useful introduction to research, the relevant concepts and its importance for developing practice. The book by Ellis, although written for nursing students, has relevance for midwifery students.

Cluett, E R and Bluff, R (eds) (2006) *Principles and practice of midwifery research* (2nd edition). Edinburgh: Elsevier.

Ellis, P (2010) *Understanding research for nursing students*. Exeter: Learning Matters.

Rees, C (2011) *Introduction to research for midwives* (3rd edition). London: Churchill Livingstone.

Ross, T (2012) *A survival guide for health research methods*. Maidenhead: McGraw-Hill.

Steen, M and Roberts, T (2011) *The handbook of midwifery research*. Oxford: Wiley.

The following are the research sources Paul looked at to develop his thinking about the third stage of labour in one of the case studies in this chapter.

Andersson, O, Hellström-Westas, L, Andersson, D and Domellöf, M (2011) Effect of delayed versus early umbilical cord clamping on neonatal outcomes and iron status at 4 months: a randomised controlled trial. *British Medical Journal*, 343: d7157.

Begley, C M, Gyte, G M L, Devane, D, McGuire, W and Weeks, A (2011) Active versus expectant management for women in the third stage of labour. *Cochrane Database of Systematic Reviews*, Issue 11. Art. No. CD007412.

Part Three

Chapter 9
Becoming a research-informed student

This chapter will help you to meet the Quality Assurance Agency for Higher Education (QAA, 2008) requirement that students studying at Level 6 are able to:

- demonstrate a systematic understanding of key aspects of their field of study, including acquisition of coherent and detailed knowledge, at least some of which is at, or informed by, the forefront of defined aspects of a discipline;
- demonstrate an ability to deploy accurately established techniques of analysis and enquiry within a discipline;
- demonstrate conceptual understanding that enables the student to describe and comment upon particular aspects of current research, or equivalent advanced scholarship, in the discipline;
- demonstrate an appreciation of the uncertainty, ambiguity and limits of knowledge;
- demonstrate the ability to manage their own learning, and to make use of scholarly reviews and primary sources (for example, refereed research articles and/or original materials appropriate to the discipline).
- critically evaluate arguments, assumptions, abstract concepts and data (that may be incomplete), to make judgements, and to frame appropriate questions to achieve a solution – or identify a range of solutions – to a problem.

NMC Standards for Pre-registration Midwifery Education

This chapter will address the following competencies:

Domain: Effective midwifery practice

Determine and provide programmes of care and support for women which:

- are based on best evidence and clinical judgment.

Provide seamless care and, where appropriate, interventions, in partnership with women and other care providers during the antenatal period which:

- are evidence based.

continued . . .

These will include:

• ensuring that current research findings and other evidence are incorporated into practice.

Work in partnership with women and other care providers during the postnatal period to provide seamless care and interventions which:

• are evidence based.

Contribute to enhancing the health and social wellbeing of individuals and their communities. This will include:

• informing practice using the best evidence which is shown to prevent and reduce maternal and perinatal morbidity and mortality.

Domain: Achieving quality care through evaluation and research
Apply relevant knowledge to the midwife's own practice in structured ways which are capable of evaluation. This will include:

• critical appraisal of knowledge and research evidence;
• disseminating critically appraised good practice.

Chapter aims

After reading this chapter you will be able to:

• use the tools of critical analysis in relation to a piece of midwifery research;
• appreciate how to critically apply research knowledge to midwifery practice.

Introduction

In the previous chapter we explored some aspects of midwifery research, and considered how research might inform midwifery practice. We then focused on the ways research is conducted and what this might indicate about the knowledge it produces. The purpose of this chapter is to provide guidance on becoming a research-informed student and practitioner. We will do this by raising awareness of the significance of ethics in midwifery research and considering midwifery research in an academically more sophisticated way, developing some of the themes already discussed. First, we will explore how to critically evaluate research, recognising that research can be a contested issue, incorporating ethical issues, and building on the understanding of critical analysis developed in Chapter 5. Using this approach, we will then consider how research can be used to inform your midwifery practice.

Critically analysing research

A reminder of critical analysis

In Chapter 5 we noted the ingredients of critical analysis. Those that are particularly relevant to critical analysis of midwifery research are:

- taking a questioning and sceptical stance;
- identifying and challenging assumptions;
- aiming for a deep understanding of knowledge and complex ideas, including an appreciation of how knowledge has been constructed;
- examining in detail different aspects of an issue;
- breaking something into its component parts;
- looking at something from different perspectives;
- recognising the role of self, and the significance of feelings, and taking a critical approach towards your own process of thinking (also linked to reflection, discussed in Chapter 7);
- being able to make an informed judgement.

Just as there are discussions about the nature of midwifery research, as highlighted in the previous chapter, so the issue of what constitutes good-quality research in midwifery is key. Writers tend to agree that midwifery research should have as its aim the improvement of maternity services in order to *maximise the capacity of women to give birth to healthy babies, to parent effectively and to build positive societies* (Downe, 2012, p14). So research should be relevant to the work of midwives – of use to the concerns of the profession. However, in order for it to be judged adequate to inform practice, it should also be conducted in a way that meets demanding academic standards of consistency and thoroughness and is methodologically sound. Both NICE and the Cochrane Library place emphasis on the need for research to meet these requirements. Wickham (2006) emphasises the importance of appraisal or evaluation of research – deciding on the value and whether it is going to be useful. She highlights two main areas of focus for such an evaluation – the methodology and the philosophy.

Ethics and research

An additional and important aspect of research that we have not yet considered and that is crucial in making a judgement about research is the ethical base of the study. Research ethics are one aspect of research governance, which provides a code for the maintenance, enhancement and monitoring of the quality of research. In midwifery research ethical criteria must normally be met before research can proceed. These are:

- non-maleficence: not doing any harm to the subjects of the research;
- beneficence: providing some benefit to those being researched;
- autonomy: respecting choice;
- justice and respect for the dignity of the individual;
- veracity: telling the truth;
- fidelity: ensuring there is trust between researcher and participants;

- positive contribution to knowledge: ensuring professional standards; using appropriate research design, methodology, methods and analysis; reporting results honestly; not falsifying results; being open about difficulties.

Universities and healthcare Trusts have their own research governance frameworks. All staff and students must gain research approval from the governance committee before they have permission to proceed with a research project. Consideration will be given to:

- purpose of study;
- design of study;
- potential benefits and risks;
- sampling procedure;
- informed consent of participants;
- data protection;
- confidentiality and anonymity;
- dissemination of findings.

When applying for ethical approval researchers will need to explain the implications of meeting the ethical code for their particular research (Cluett and Bluff, 2006; Ellis, 2010).

Activity 9.1   *Research and finding out*

Research ethics

Locate a copy of the code of ethics for research for your university.

Read it through carefully. Identify the aspects that you think are of most importance to midwifery research.

Comment

You might have identified the following.

- Because midwifery research could involve women and families in vulnerable situations, the meaning of *informed consent* to the research might need very careful consideration.
- Since research might lead to the sharing of sensitive information, *confidentiality* should be thought about in depth.

Any critical analysis of midwifery research must integrate an understanding of the ethics of research, as outlined next.

Critical analysis of research: a framework

In your studies at Level 6 you will be expected to use midwifery research in order to develop a full and specialist understanding of a topic and to guide your thinking and practice. This will mean both being able to approach research in a critical way and being able to identify its strengths and weaknesses and potential for informing practice. The questions set out below provide a framework that can be used to evaluate a piece of research.

Research topic

- Is the research well informed by the existing knowledge base?
- Has it drawn on a good range of the existing literature on the topic?
- Is the research an appropriate development of existing knowledge?
- Does the research have a focus on improving services for women?

Research question(s)

- What were the question(s) the research set out to answer?
- Are the question(s) well thought out and clear?
- Is the selection of research question(s) adequately argued and justified?

Research ethics

- Are the research ethics clearly set out?
- Are all relevant aspects of research ethics considered?
- Are there ethical considerations that have been overlooked?
- Are there ethical dilemmas that have not been explored?
- How was the research funded and are there any possible implications?

The conduct of the research

- How was the research carried out?
- Is the methodology clear? Is it appropriate to the topic and the research questions?
- Is the design of the research well thought out?
- What methods were used to collect the data? Are they clear and appropriate to the topic?
- Is the way the data was analysed clear and justified?

Findings

- What are the main conclusions to be drawn from the research?
- Are the claims of the implications of the findings consistent with the aims of the research and the methodology?
- Have the difficulties of the research been outlined and discussed?
- Is the research realistic about negative or neutral results?
- What contribution does the research make to the overall knowledge of the topic?
- What contribution might the research make to midwifery practice?

Reflection

- How do I feel about the research topic, the way it has been carried out and the findings?
- Why might I have responded to the research in this way?
- What are the implications of this for my thinking about the topic?
- What is the impact on my judgements about the research?

Overall

- What conclusions can I draw about the value of this research?
- In summary, what is the justification for this conclusion?
- How might this guide practice ?

These questions make a rather long list, and when considering pieces of research you may not answer every question. For instance, you may be reading a shortened account of the research in a journal article, rather than the whole research study, and this may mean that not all the issues you wish to explore are discussed. However, it will assist your critical analysis skills if you aim to cover all these points.

Activity 9.2   *Critical thinking*

Critically analysing research

Select an article from *Evidence Based Midwifery* or *British Journal of Midwifery* on a topic that is relevant to your current practice placement. Read it through once to get a general understanding. Then read it again using the questions above in order to develop a critical analysis.

Case study: Paul analyses some research on stillbirths

While Paul was on his third-year placement on a labour ward he became interested in assumptions that were made about two stillbirths that occurred during his time there. He had overheard comments such as 'Well, of course, she smoked all through the pregnancy', and this prompted him to reflect on whether this direct causal link was valid. Keen to find evidence, he looked for relevant research. One article in particular reported recent findings that he felt could be useful. His module leader, Kate, reminded him that he should take a critically analytic approach to his reading. Below we can see some of Paul's thinking, which developed using the framework for analysis above. It is presented in note form but should enable you to see some results of critical analysis. You might also find it helpful to read the article for yourself.

Gardosi, J, Madurasinghe, V, Williams, S, Malik, A and Francis, A (2013) Maternal and fetal risk factors for stillbirth: population based study *British Medical Journal*, 346: f108.

Research topic

- The article builds on existing research referred to through footnotes. If I wanted to develop my understanding for a more extended university assignment, these would be useful sources to draw on.

- The authors observe that previously risk factors have been thought to be poor predictors of stillbirth and they wished to look further at this.
- Because stillbirth rates in the UK are relatively high compared to countries with similar income levels, this is an important and justifiable piece of research. It has also helped me to evaluate views I have heard in practice.
- The article notes that parent-led campaigns have emphasised the need for more work to be done in the prevention of stillbirth. Hence the article makes a useful contribution to the reduction of both physical and emotional distress for women and their families.

Research question(s)

- The research questions were as follows.
  - i) What are the demographic, social and medical risk factors for stillbirth that can be ascertained at the beginning of pregnancy, or become apparent as the pregnancy progresses, in a multi-ethnic English maternity population?
  - ii) What is the contribution of these to stillbirth?
- The research questions were clear and well focused, and a sound justification for them was provided.

Research ethics

- The article sets out the arrangements for confidentiality and consent. The confidentiality of individual women was assured by giving them pseudonyms. This seems sound. An account of how maternal consent was obtained, and the possibility of opt-out, is provided. However, it does not explain the ways in which truly informed consent was assured. This may be because of article length restrictions in an academic journal. But I wonder whether prospective mothers might have felt pressure to agree to their data being used – particularly at a time of hopefulness and expectation of a live birth.
- Other aspects of research ethics are not set out in the article – however, the research seems to conform to relevant principles. In particular, I consider that it has the potential to make a positive contribution to knowledge, and the research design supports this.
- The data collection and analytic staff were financially supported by NHS West Midlands Strategic Health Authority and all the relevant primary care Trusts. The researchers, who were employed by research departments, made a declaration that the funders had no influence on the design, writing up or submission for publication of the research. They also declared that there were no competing interests or activities/interests that could appear to have influenced the

completed work. So, as far as is possible, the research would seem to be free of any pressure exerted by financial sponsors.

The conduct of the research

- The research was carried out through the collection and analysis of data.
- The methodology is quantitative: a large cohort study of 92,218 normally formed single pregnancies including 389 stillbirths from 24 weeks' gestation, delivered between 2009 and 2011. The methodology is clearly set out and well justified. The numbers involved give the research weight, and the multi-ethnic population ensures that a range of social and economic factors were explored for relevance.
- The research design is thorough and appropriate to the research questions. Criteria and definitions are thought through and justified – for example, the criterion of including only normally formed singletons – thus excluding congenital abnormalities from the cohort.
- The data was collected from existing documents – hand-held maternity notes kept by midwives – between 2009 and 2011. Information was transferred from the notes to electronic records at the end of pregnancy. Quality and consistency was said to be assured through training and audits. A data set of 87 items of information, theorised as relevant to stillbirth, were noted. The article does not consider the possibility of these items being missing from maternity notes or of the data clerks missing crucial items through human error. The researchers provide academic validation for the use of their indicators of intra-uterine growth restriction and foetal growth restriction.
- The data analysis was complex. Statistical techniques used were univariate and then multivariate analysis using a regression model. The aim was to explore the impact of a range of variables, and the relationship between them, on stillbirth. A statistical package STATA version 11 was used to do this. This approach and the package used have academic respectability. In order to more fully understand the statistical approaches used, I referred to a helpful book – Salkind, N J (2011) *Statistics for people who (think they) hate statistics*. London: Sage.
- The findings described in the text of the article are set out in tables, which enable the reader to follow them in depth and detail.

Findings

- The main finding of the research was that, together, maternal obesity, smoking and fetal growth restriction are modifiable risk factors found in 56.1 per cent of cases of normally formed stillbirths. The single most important risk factor was found to be unrecognised fetal growth restriction. The highest risk of stillbirth was in pregnancies with fetal growth restriction where the mother did not smoke.

However, the authors argue that because there is a known association between smoking and fetal growth restriction, there is a possibility that potential risks, such as non-smoking mothers subject to passive smoking, are missed. The term 'history of mental health problems' is used without definition, and I wondered how broadly this was applied. I also looked up 'modifiable risk factor' and learnt that it means factors that can be controlled, or treated. Given the complexity of issues such as smoking and obesity, I felt there were unwarranted assumptions about what can be treated and controlled and the effectiveness of current interventions. At present low birth weight cannot be controlled or treated – it can only be monitored – and, if there are concerns, early delivery can be planned.

- I had a few questions about the researchers' confidence in their conclusions. While a statistical correlation was clearly made, I wonder if there was a danger of this being seen as causal. There were some factors the researchers considered – e.g. alcohol consumption and use of non-prescription drugs (and possibly smoking) – that, when the notes were made, would rely on self-report. These issues tend to be under-reported. So the incidence of these and their impact might be underplayed in the results.

- The claims that most normally formed singleton stillbirths are avoidable seemed to me to be ambitious. The researchers argue for improving current strategies and protocols for improved surveillance of fetal growth during the antenatal period.

- The authors note one limitation: that consent rates for post-mortem examinations among some ethnic groups are low and so some undiagnosed congenital abnormalities might have been included in the cohort, thus skewing the risk factor for those groups.

- The research has added to an understanding of risk factors in stillbirth and alerted midwifery to an aspect of practice that could be given more attention.

- The research suggests that midwives should be more alert to fetal growth restriction especially when it has not traditionally been anticipated, e.g. in the instance of non-smoking mothers. It is less specific about what can then be done to prevent stillbirth.

Reflection

- I felt the research was helpful in exploring risk factors that related to stillbirth although in many ways it raised more questions than it answered – which is often true of research. In my experience stillbirth is an extremely distressing and emotional event, and it felt a little odd that this was not really reflected in the academic way the research was presented. I think I have learnt that midwives need to operate in different ways at different times: when involved in a stillbirth you need sensitivity, empathy, carefulness and to be able to manage your feelings so you can be helpful to the woman and her family; but you also need to be able to put on your 'thinking' head so that you can use valid evidence as a means of improving practice.

- I have participated in, and observed, antenatal assessment by midwives of fetal growth – using their hands and eyes and measuring tape. The NICE Antenatal Guidelines (2008) recommend symphysis–fundal height measurement with tape, and the full guidelines include a useful discussion on the effectiveness of this. When my mentors have had concerns about apparent lack of fetal growth they have referred women for additional obstetric assessment, ultrasound (USS) and consultant check-ups. This has sometimes identified poor growth and resulted in an induction and closer monitoring in labour. Mostly USS has suggested normal growth, but sometimes women have found the process of referral unsettling. I can see there is a need for further research on how clinicians can assess fetal growth in more consistent and effective ways.

Overall

- Overall I consider this research useful and will incorporate its findings into my thinking about risk. My hope is that I will also be able to use it to be more alert in my practice with women antenatally. I plan to look out for new research on the topic to see if it draws similar conclusions.

Critical application to practice

We now move to thinking in more detail about how research might guide midwifery practice. In order to assist this we provide a series of pointers towards becoming a research informed student and an example of using research in practice.

Becoming research informed

In your particular area of midwifery practice, develop the habits of:

- being enquiring about and alert to what research is currently available;
- regularly checking websites and keeping up to date;
- focusing on reliable and relevant sources;
- using research guidance and reviews.

In relation to specific topics or issues:

- search thoroughly: you may need to use various search terms to find what you need;
- access and read a range of material;
- be alert to the historical relevance and/or currency of the material.

In dealing with what you find:

- consider pieces of research in relation to others;
- take a critically analytic approach (as outlined above);
- try to identify whether the research study might relate to your specific and individual issue;
- consider whether the research material helps you to look at the situation differently;
- ask whether, and in what ways, the research might lead you to practise in a particular way.

Activity 9.3   *Research and finding out*

Becoming research-informed

Think of a practice issue in your current placement about which you wanted to know more or about which you had some uncertainties. Use the above approach to discover how research might provide some helpful indicators.

Case study: Linda's third-year placement and becoming research informed

Linda had now observed and been involved in births in different settings: in women's homes; on a labour ward; and in a midwife-led birth centre. She wanted to find out more about what difference the setting might make to the mother and her child.

She had assisted with one birth on a labour ward that had seemed very relaxed for both the parents and the baby and another birth where the environment did not seem to be conducive to the father feeling welcomed or to provide the opportunity for the mother and baby to bond. From her own experiences of giving birth, Linda thought that the most important factors for her had been her trust in the midwives and her relationships with them. But on reflection she appreciated that her local maternity hospital had been recently refitted, and the birthing rooms were spacious and well decorated with their own bathrooms, in order to enhance privacy. Looking back, she could not remember anyone mentioning the idea of having a home birth.

Below is an example of how Linda used the approach outlined above to help her develop her research informed thinking about the significance of the place of birth.

Awareness of existing research

As part of Linda's preparation for her midwifery course she had read several midwifery journal articles and looked at internet information-sharing sites. She had wanted to increase her background knowledge of issues that were important for women and the key things that made midwives want to do the job. Place of birth and the environment of birth had seemed very important. Now she had experience of observing how a careful and nurturing approach from midwives could overcome many physical problems, but she knew from her most recent course reading and learning that place of birth is a central pillar of midwifery practice. It is also a politically sensitive issue in planning for service provision and central government policy and legislation, with considerable debate about safety versus choice.

continued ...

Linda looked at her reading list and used this as a starting point for finding relevant studies that might help her to build a clearer picture. Here are some of her findings.

Classic texts from midwifery literature and historical statistics

- *The original work on safety and place of birth produced by lecturer Marjorie Tew dates from the late 1970s when she was teaching medical students and found she had to challenge the analysis of the government statistics. When the data was carefully and accurately analysed for the first time, she found clear evidence that home birth posed no higher risks for low-risk women (Tew, 1998).*

- *Mary Cronk, writing with the benefit of decades of midwifery practice, points out some well-intentioned motivations that formed part of the drive towards hospital birth in the 1960s and 1970s. Poverty, poor housing and lack of basic facilities made home birth difficult for mothers and the midwives, who often had to work hard to get higher-risk women into hospitals (Cronk and Jowitt, 1997). Linda had also read some published experiences of midwives working at that time and was amazed to read how midwives coped at home births where there were outside toilets and no running water (Dunn, 2010; Worth, 2008).*

- *Having previously explored Nicky Leap's (1996) work, Linda had often seen the Albany Group Practice – led by her, Jane Sandall and Jane Grant – referenced. However, she had not realised that this pioneering NHS-funded group worked with mainly disadvantaged women and that the choice of where to have the baby was generally made in labour in the woman's home. She was surprised to see that 66 per cent of women who used the services of the practice in 1995 had chosen to have a home birth. The way in which midwives at the Albany shared information and kept the focus on community care, together with the women's own family and support network, appeared key in making choices.*

Two reviews on the Cochrane database about place of birth that summarise some of the key issues from good quality research papers

- *Alternative versus conventional institutional settings for birth (Hodnett et al., 2012). The objectives of this review were to compare the effects of care in an alternative institutional birth environment with those in a conventional setting and to determine if such effects are influenced by staffing, architectural features, organisational models or geographical location. The review concluded that hospital birth centres were associated with lower rates of medical interventions during labour and birth, and higher levels of satisfaction without increasing risk to either mothers or babies.*

- *Planned hospital birth versus planned home birth (Olsen and Clausen, 2012). This review aimed to assess the effects of planned hospital birth compared with planned home birth in selected low-risk women, assisted by an experienced midwife with collaborative medical back-up in case transfer should be necessary. Linda found this in-depth analysis of all the factors to be considered when looking at risk and birth particularly valuable. The review covered only randomised control trials so it did not include the results of the Birthplace Study (Brocklehurst et al., 2011), which Linda read next.*

Department of Health research and government policy

- *Brocklehurst et al. (2011): Linda knew that this important Birthplace in England Collaborative Group research study had considered risk and safety in relation to home birth for lower-risk women. It found that women planning birth in a midwifery unit and multiparous women planning birth at home experience*

continued . . .

fewer interventions than those planning birth in an obstetric unit, and that this lower intervention rate has had no impact on perinatal outcomes. She was also interested to read in a related article that home birth appeared to be more cost-effective in terms of service provision for multiparous women (Schroeder et al., 2012).

- *The Department of Health's* Maternity matters *(DH, 2007) outlined the changes ahead for the funding and planning of maternity services. These included the provision of choice for women on place of birth: a home birth, a hospital birth or birth in a midwifery-led unit. This led Linda to some online research of her own on how Trusts were complying with these targets.*

Women's experience of transfer in labour

Linda followed up her earlier interest in transfer in labour by reading additional articles. Rowe et al. (2012a) found that women with higher risks of transfer included nulliparous women under 20 years, women over 35, those starting labour care after 40 weeks of gestation and the presence of complicating conditions at the start of labour care. Rowe et al. (2012b) made uncomfortable reading but gave Linda some real insights into how sensitive information can be delivered, the importance of clear handover and consideration for the feelings of the woman and family at all times.

Statistics on place of birth

Linda did not find it easy to access current figures about place of birth from her own Trust. National government figures were easier to find on the internet, and she could see a variation in rates across England and Wales (Office for National Statistics, accessed 2012). The BirthChoice UK site (accessed 2013) yielded the same information but provided easier links to make comparisons between Trusts and to access women's experience of care from a Care Quality Commission Survey (CQC, 2010). Home birth rates between 1 per cent and 3 per cent were the most common, but in some regions rates were higher. Linda had read about home birth initiatives in Wales and thought that the figures of 5.7 per cent and 4.2 per cent in some Welsh districts might reflect their impact. However, these national statistics did not differentiate between planned and unplanned home births.

The voices of women and consumer groups

- *Having looked at the views of women surveyed by the Care Quality Commission (CQC, 2010) and the National Perinatal Epidemiological (NPEU) report on women's experience of maternity care (Redshaw and Heikka, 2010), Linda could see that there was a variation in how women were offered information and their expectations of service provision. She was surprised to see that 80 per cent of women surveyed in the NPEU study – a very high figure – were not made aware of the possible options for place of birth as stipulated in* Maternity matters *(DH, 2007). Although she found a large amount of literature on what women valued in terms of midwifery care and their experience of birth in different settings, there was comparatively little that asked women directly what they wanted in relation to place of birth.*
- *On a local level, Linda discussed with other students in her study group how the views of women about place of birth and choices within the Trust could be found. Her group decided to find out what was available. One student looked at websites and social network sites such as Mumsnet and another researched the National Childbirth Trust and Maternity Services Liaison Committees (MSLC). When the group*

continued . . .

pooled their findings the local picture was mixed. Local mothers and support groups were involved with the local Maternity Services Liaison Committee, but information gleaned from the Trust's website did not make it clear what had been learnt about women's views on place of birth. There were attempts by the Trust to gain feedback and views through hospital questionnaires, feedback boxes and the Patient Advice and Liaison Service (PALS), but the group could not find any reports on findings that were specific to maternity issues such as place of birth. Linda learnt that the local midwives supervisors' group had made efforts to support women to make choices regarding place of birth and had displayed posters in practice areas and children's centres about the options available. She decided to contact the supervision team to find out how they contributed to feeding back information to the Trust and to future policy development.

From all this Linda concluded the following

- *She was much clearer about the findings of the research. For example, she found it helpful to appreciate the way in which safety is discussed and measured in relation to place of birth (Brocklehurst et al., 2011). From reading the review by Hodnett et al. (2012) she could now more confidently explain that birth centres were a safe choice for low-risk women and associated with higher levels of satisfaction for women.*
- *Linda felt that looking at original pieces of research or literature and then at reviews had helped her to really think about factors that might complicate direct comparisons between different settings for birth. Confounders – issues that could blur direct comparisons of effect and outcome between two variables or two birth settings – could include: differences in the organisations involved; the models of care, i.e. how staffing is organised; continuity of carer; and the social class and possible psychological advantages of those who exercise choices.*
- *The predominant emphasis in the research is on physical safety. Linda felt that all midwives would need to consider how to respond to the findings from the Birthplace Study regarding risk of home birth for babies of first-time mothers. However, the risks and safety of hospital birth, particularly for multiparous women with straightforward pregnancies, needed more exploration.*
- *Where babies are born is a long-standing political and feminist issue, and debate around it seems likely to continue.*
- *Women's views about place of birth are often implied in the literature without validation by research. Linda was surprised about the profound effect that the availability of choices, and how these are presented to women, had on take-up.*

Linda's research-informed practice

Linda decided she would use her learning from this to focus more on careful listening and clear, relevant information-giving when discussing the possibilities for women around place of birth. She had begun to develop these skills from her mentors in practice. However, the research literature had alerted her to the high expectations placed on the clinician by women and the importance of how questions and answers were worded. She decided to concentrate on learning some of the statistical findings from the Birthplace Study so that she could be confident in the information that she was sharing. Linda also planned to find out more about place of birth in relation to her own Trust. What statistics were available currently and from where? What were the Trust's policies for safeguarding choice in the immediate future? She also hoped to develop the topic of transfer in labour for her dissertation.

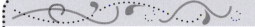

Chapter summary

In this chapter we have built on Chapter 8 to use higher-level academic skills in relation to research. We began with a discussion about the ethics of research and their significance in both carrying out and evaluating research. The tools for critical analysis of research were provided and demonstrated through Paul examining a piece of research on stillbirth. We next considered how research might inform midwifery practice, and a set of pointers together with an example from Linda's studies were presented. While the focus of the chapter has been on research, it is important to remember that research is not the only factor to take into account when thinking about practice. It will need to be weighed up and incorporated with other factors when exploring a topic or planning midwifery practice interventions. In Chapters 11 and 12 we will include research findings along with theory, knowledge and values to appreciate the complexity of midwifery thinking and practice.

Further reading

Steen, M and Roberts, T (2011*) The handbook of midwifery research.* Oxford: Wiley.

A useful guide to midwifery research, particularly the sections on searching and making sense of research.

Wickham, S (2006) *Appraising research into childbirth.* London: Elsevier.

Sarah Wickham provides worked examples of appraising research, looking at topics such as women's views, women's experiences and childbirth interventions.

Chapter 10
Becoming an independent and autonomous learner

This chapter will help you to meet the Quality Assurance Agency for Higher Education (QAA, 2008) requirement that students studying at Level 6 are able to:

- demonstrate the ability to manage their own learning, and to make use of scholarly reviews and primary sources (for example, refereed research articles and/or original materials appropriate to the discipline);
- apply the methods and techniques that they have learned to review, consolidate, extend and apply their knowledge and understanding, and to initiate and carry out projects.

Students at this level will also have the learning ability needed to undertake appropriate further training of a professional or equivalent nature.

NMC Standards for Pre-registration Midwifery Education

This chapter will address the following competencies:

Domain: Developing the individual midwife and others
Review, develop and enhance the midwife's own knowledge, skills and fitness to practise. This will include:

- making effective use of the framework for the statutory supervision of midwives;
- meeting the NMC's continuing professional development and practice standards;
- reflecting on the midwife's own practice and making the necessary changes as a result;
- attending conferences, presentations and other learning events.

Contribute to the audit of practice in order to optimise the care of women, babies and their families. This will include:

- auditing the individual's own practice;
- contributing to the audit of team practice.

> **Chapter aims**
>
> After reading this chapter you will be able to:
>
> • appreciate how to become a more independent learner;
> • reflect on and identify how you learn;
> • understand the importance of, and your role in, continuing professional development.

Introduction

When you are studying at Level 6 of a degree, it is expected that the process, as well as the content, of your learning will be different and more complex. So it is important to give some attention to how you are studying. As you progress through the degree you should become aware of how you learn so that you are able to manage your own learning more fully – becoming an autonomous and independent learner. This means that you are able to self-direct your learning, needing less guidance, teaching and support. Another aspect of being an independent learner is appreciating that achieving the degree is one stage in your **continuing professional development**, which will be part of being a midwife. Taking an active role in this means being able to identify your future learning needs. This awareness of and reflection on how you learn, appreciation of your learning needs and ability to respond appropriately is known as meta-cognition. In this chapter different aspects of metacognition will be explored.

Becoming an independent learner

On your course the assignments and learning activities will be designed to support you in moving towards independence in learning so that by the final year you should be self-directing and autonomous. In particular when you are working on your final project or dissertation, there is an expectation that you will work with a high level of independence. Here we will identify the attributes of an independent and autonomous learner, and consider the value of reflection in moving towards an understanding of both how you learn and areas for developmental growth.

> **Activity 10.1**   *Reflection*
>
> **The characteristics of an independent and autonomous learner**
>
> List what you think are the characteristics of an independent and autonomous learner. Then compare your list with the points in the research summary below.

Research summary: the characteristics of an independent and autonomous learner

Taking responsibility for your own learning: Taking charge of your own learning and acting independently; being less reliant on tutors and classes for your learning; not using as much guidance and support; recognising that you learn in a different way from other people, so you will need to choose your own direction, formulate your own problems and decide on your course of action.

Having an engaged disposition towards learning and understanding learning as an active process: not passively receiving and reproducing material but engaging with ideas, identifying relationships and interconnections; building on what you know, interpreting, restructuring and transforming your understanding as you learn more; appreciating that you will need to put mental effort into making personal sense of new information and experiences; seeing learning as continuous, ongoing and lifelong.

Actively participating in supervision and tutorials: thinking ahead to supervision and tutorials, identifying the guidance and direction you need; being prepared with questions, issues, ideas and suggestions; actively contributing to discussion and debate.

Using feedback, both positive and negative: carefully reading and assimilating feedback; ensuring you understand what it means; allowing yourself to be challenged by it; working out what you need to do as a result and implementing this.

Setting your own learning goals: being clear about your long-term objectives; identifying short-term goals that will help you work towards the objectives; monitoring your progress towards meeting the goals; making adjustments if necessary.

Developing key study skills and strategies that work for you: for example, managing time; developing strategies for reading or writing.

Being self-monitoring: knowing what are effective ways of studying for you; being able to develop your own learning strategies; being able to self-assess your progress.

Discovering your own learning resources: independently exploring sources of knowledge and research; being able to make informed judgements about the value of resources.

Seeking out, being alert to and recognising learning opportunities: in university, on your placement and in other aspects of your life.

Being self-aware and self-evaluating: learning to judge and evaluate your own thinking and writing to develop creativity and self-reliance; being able to identify your own progress in learning.

Academic assertiveness: developing your own 'voice' in debates; being able to challenge and be challenged; recovering from situations of failure; being open to feedback; being able to listen to other viewpoints; being able to make and justify independent viewpoints having realistic confidence and self-esteem.

Personal motivation to achieve your aim: having intellectual curiosity about the subject; seeing the goal as worthwhile; valuing the tasks that contribute towards the goal.

(Biggs, 2003; Chan, 2001; Clare, 2007; Eraut, 1994; Gibbs, 1981; Gordon and Cooper, 2010; Macaulay, 2000; McMillan, 2010; Moon, 2008; Race, 2010)

This is an ambitious list of the characteristics of the ideal learner. However, all these attributes will tend to feed into and reinforce each other, thereby developing your capacity to learn. Working on one should support the development of others. Many of these attributes are transferable to midwifery practice and the characteristics expected of a professional practitioner.

Activity 10.2   *Reflection*

Self-evaluation

Looking at the list above, evaluate yourself as an independent and autonomous learner. Think about this in relation to both university and your placement. Identify areas for development.

Case study: Nazneen's self-evaluation

At the first tutorial for her dissertation, Nazneen was asked by her tutor to think about how far she had progressed as an independent learner. Below is her self-evaluation using the headings set out above.

Taking responsibility for your own learning: *From where I started on the course, having achieved A levels, I have needed to learn to rely less on the instructions and guidance of teachers and think much more about what and how I need to learn in order to become a competent midwife.*

Having an active disposition towards learning and understanding learning as an active process: *When I am mulling things over in my mind (often on the bus coming home from university) I am relating the teaching to my experiences on placement. And it works the other way round too. My whole attitude towards learning has changed. I really work at trying to make sense of things. My boyfriend teases me about this – I question everything now.*

Actively participating in supervision and tutorials: *I was very nervous in tutorials at first and thought I would learn more by listening to other people. But I have gradually become more confident and have discovered that, by asking questions and trying out ideas with others, my thinking has really developed.*

Using feedback both positive and negative: *I have found it difficult to read feedback on assignments – really because I was so scared that it would challenge me in a way that would make me feel inadequate. Since I began taking a deep breath and sitting quietly to read, and think about, how the feedback might help me develop, I have found it easier. Now I can see how feedback can 'feed forward' to the next assignment or task.*

Setting your own learning goals: *Again, I have been reluctant to do this for myself – really wanting someone else (who knows more than me) to do this. However, I can see the importance of working methodically and to targets – and to set them for myself. For my dissertation I will draw up a time plan for the whole piece of work with short-term and long-term goals.*

Developing key study skills and strategies which work for you: *I am still working on this. When I started the course I was so focused on the goal of getting a qualification that I used study skills that got the*

continued . . .

work done on time but did not always develop my learning. Then I went the other way. My aim for the dissertation is to find a better balance.

Being self-monitoring: *I am getting better at working out how I study best, not doing what my family suggest but seeing what has really helped me to develop. I have had to change some aspects of how I learn and do things I would not have anticipated, such as taking notes and using a highlighter.*

Discovering your own learning resources: *I now love spending time searching for resources. There is a risk that I can get carried away and not always use my time well. It has taken me a while to be able to work out the relative value of different sources of research and information. I need to work on this, especially for my dissertation.*

Seeking out, being alert to and recognising learning opportunities: *This has been a big shift for me – it feels as if I can hardly stop learning.*

Being self-aware and self-evaluating: *I am making progress, but there is room for development here. I think I could be more rigorous. My tendency is still to leave it to lecturers and my practice assessors to highlight the weaknesses in my work.*

Academic assertiveness: *I think I am finding my own particular contribution to discussions and debates and seeing that others appreciate the different perspective I sometimes bring because I come from an Asian family. My new, more balanced, grasp of my strengths and weaknesses provides me with a sounder base from which to make judgements. It has been important for me to go through this process as a student, professionally and personally. My friends and family outside the course sometimes seem a little startled by my new confidence. But they also quite like it.*

Personal motivation to achieve your aim: *I was always passionate about becoming a midwife, doing midwifery, and this has helped me through the difficult parts of the course. What's more, I can really see now how the thinking and reflecting side of it is important – and I have come to love that too. My interest in grasping concepts, looking at issues from different perspectives and exploring all sides of a problem, has definitely grown. As my approach to learning has shifted I can appreciate the purpose of the classroom activities and assignments, and their relevance to learning and to becoming a midwife.*

Metacognition

One way of making progress as an independent learner is to develop your skills in metacognition. This means:

- conscious awareness of your own learning capacity and your experience of learning;
- your ability to articulate this – being able to explain how you have learnt and transformed your understanding;
- using this to monitor and adjust your approach to learning and problem solving – to choose, revise or abandon learning strategies.
  (Eraut, 1994; Jackson, 2004; Moon, 2005; Stephenson, 2001).

Writers on learners and learning suggest that metacognition is not possible without a deep approach to learning as discussed in Chapter 1 (Marshall and Case, 2005). Nazneen's thoughtfulness about her learning (above) demonstrates that she is developing her skills of metacognition; she recognises her own knowledge together with processes of, and strategies for, knowing.

In Chapter 7 we considered the value of reflection in developing your midwifery practice. Here we are using reflection for a slightly different purpose – to understand and develop your metacognition. Moon (2004, 2005) suggests that you need to be able to stand back from yourself and not think about what you have learnt but, rather, think about the cognitive processes. This might mean reflecting on how you tackled a task, what are the ingredients when things are going well, what is going on when they are not – and why. Fonteyn and Cahill (1998) report on research with nursing students that suggests that the use of reflective clinical logs at the end of a shift improved their ability *to think about their thinking* (p149).

In Chapter 7 the significance of the impact of our emotions was noted as an important aspect of reflection on practice. Similarly, in reflection on learning, the role of feelings must be considered for they connect to your motivation, your mood and your level of self-worth. All of these will impact on how you learn.

Activity 10.3   *Critical thinking*

One way of reflecting on learning

Identify one learning experience. For example: writing an assignment in which you were asked to make a judgement; researching literature to understand an issue in more depth; engaging in a debate in university; or using theory on placement to inform how to work with a woman.

Describe the learning experience using the following questions.

- What happened?
- What were the main components of the experience?

This is the *content* of the experience. To really engage in reflection you need to move on to thinking about the *process* of the experience. Reflect on how you learnt using these questions.

- What was I trying to achieve?
- Why did I go about it in the way I did?
- How was I feeling? What impact did this have?
- How did my previous experiences of learning affect how I felt and what I did?
- How successful was this learning?
- What factors helped to make this successful?
- What was the impact of the way I went about this?
- What other choices did I have?
- What might have been the consequences of the other choices?

continued . . . ●●

Learning from the experience, you could ask yourself these questions.

- How do I feel now about the experience?
- Could I have dealt with it differently?
- What have I learnt from this that I might be able to use in new situations?
- What might get in the way of my doing things differently?

Comment

We discussed ways of developing reflection for practice in Chapter 7. Similarly, when reflecting on your learning, a journal, a **critical friend**, supervision and tutorials can all be helpful. For instance, sometimes your tutor will be able to support you in thinking about the way you have gone about a learning task. Levett-Jones (2007) suggests a particular process that she calls a nursing narrative, which sets out a structured approach for developing an in-depth analysis of, and reflection on, the meaning of the episode. She argues that the power of narrative reflection is its potential to enhance the ability to critique and learn from practice and so develop clinical competence. Through it students can articulate, appreciate and value their practice.

Moon (2004) argues that **second-order reflection** can further enhance reflection. This means taking a piece of reflective writing already completed and considering it in order to write a deeper reflective overview. By doing this you should be able to identify the impact of your attitudes towards a particular topic or the impact of particular emotional states and how these might have shifted with different understanding. In this way you can act as your own critical friend.

Case study: Linda's internet search – reflection and second-order reflection

Shortly before she started a placement in the community Linda carried out an internet search to find material on female genital mutilation for a university presentation. Afterwards Linda wrote reflectively.

I wanted to collect some literature that would help me to put together a ten-minute class presentation on female genital mutilation that I was due to give the following week. So I tried different search terms and different websites. I got either loads of hits or nothing. I had avoided working on this and focused on a different piece of work because of my anxiety about doing a presentation – but also maybe because I didn't want to think about this topic. So I ended up doing the search at home with my teenage children nagging me because they wanted to use the computer and giving me unhelpful advice about Wikipedia. This stressed me out more. My partner Gary had offered to cook the dinner, but I thought I could smell burning from the kitchen. Distracted, I kept making silly mistakes and losing my way. Previously in university I had managed searches with reasonable success – although I knew I needed more practice. In this situation I found it hard to build on the skills I had learnt and make progress.

But I think the biggest obstacle to my making progress was the topic. When we dealt with the general topic of abuse in university, we covered a number of issues. I found it very

continued . . .

upsetting. Some of the categories of abuse made me feel sick. I didn't talk to anyone about this, but I knew I was full of dread about having to explore it more. This is probably why I had left it rather late and was almost sabotaging the research by the timing and circumstances. After finding a few relevant articles I gave up, let the children use the computer and went to the kitchen where I criticised Gary's cooking and had a glass of wine. So that night I didn't sleep well because I hadn't successfully done the search and knew I shouldn't have taken it out on Gary.

Learning from the experience

I now feel a bit silly for doing what I did. After the university class I knew I had some sorting out to do in my own head. What we learnt made me think about my anxieties about my own children and how I don't understand how children can be hurt in this way. How could I possibly have started researching the topic of female genital mutilation without processing this? Even in the best of circumstances I would have struggled, and I set up for myself the worst of circumstances and nearly risked a big family upset. I also knew that I was soon to start a placement in the community in a very multicultural area, and I had wondered how I would react if I came across this issue, so my anxiety about that was high. Obviously I could, and should, have found a better time and place to carry out the search. I now feel disappointed and cross with myself – I thought I had learnt more than this on the course.

Later Linda used her 'critical friend' Maggie for some second-order reflection

A week later Linda showed Maggie what she had written. Maggie was really helpful in pointing out that when Linda wrote the account her self-esteem was low because of her disappointment with herself. She suggested that Linda was at risk of getting stuck in despair and reminded her of all the positive things she had achieved on the course. She helped Linda reframe the experience so it could be used constructively to develop Linda's learning.

Linda noted that in future she would try to be more self-aware, more conscious of her emotions and not block them. She thought that exploring her feelings could be a useful tool for learning and she needed to find an appropriate place to do this. She wondered if, by starting the search in the way she did, she had wanted unconsciously to share her upset and anxiety, which she could not communicate openly, with Gary and her children. This led on to more thinking and learning about people in distress and the many indirect ways they let other people know this. When Linda was on her placement she found this learning really helpful.

Future learning

By the end of the midwifery degree, as an independent and autonomous learner, you should be able to appreciate and articulate your learning journey. This means, first, thinking about: how far you have travelled since you began your course; what you have learnt; how you have learned to learn; your personal and professional growth; the skills and qualities you have developed. Thinking about this reflectively can be rewarding and affirming. While you are studying, the demands of the course and the need to complete the next assignment can often get in the way of taking stock, appreciating how and why you have developed. At the final stage of the course you should complete the section of the Personal Development Plan (PDP), which we first discussed in Chapter 1, to make sense of your experience and record your achievements. It can be very useful to work with a critical friend or a tutor to help you clarify your thinking, and identify your growth and development. You might find it helpful to look back to your answers to Activity 1.1 as a reminder of yourself when you started the course.

Second, you need to give some attention to the learning journey ahead of you, together with your needs and goals for continuing learning and development. When you reach the end of the course it may seem as if you have reached the end of your journey. However, for practising professionals, learning is a lifelong process – you will need to go on acquiring and updating knowledge and skills, exploring values and adapting to change. While your training and education have provided you with a qualification to work as a midwife and you will have skills and some expertise from your placement settings, this will not be sufficient for your career.

Minimum requirements for continuing professional development (CPD) set by the Nursing and Midwifery Council can be found in their guidance on post-registration education and practice (Prep) (NMC, 2011a). Midwives must:

*   practise as a midwife for a minimum of 450 hours during the three years prior to the renewal of their registration;
*   undertake at least 35 hours of learning activity relevant to their practice every three years;
*   maintain a personal professional profile of their learning activity.

The current *NHS Knowledge and Skills Framework* (DH, 2004) to support education and development within the NHS also created gateways for career progression, so midwives must demonstrate that they can apply learning and skills within their role in order to move forward to the next pay grade.

Continuing professional development has benefits additional to meeting the requirements of the NMC. It can provide a way of keeping a balanced perspective in the demanding, shifting and uncertain world of midwifery practice. It enables you to maintain contact with current research, theories and ideas. While keeping you up to date, it should also be stimulating and provide material for reflection on your practice (Eraut, 1994; Lishman, 2007).

Being able to appreciate your future learning needs is a fundamental aspect of being an autonomous learner. Thoughtfully and thoroughly completing your PDP will provide you with a record of your achievement and your future learning needs in a document you can share with current and prospective employers, and, if you choose, your supervisor of midwives, demonstrating your understanding of the importance of continuing professional development.

Activity 10.4   *Reflection*

My development as a learner

As you approach the end of the course try to summarise:

*   the personal development you have achieved through the course;
*   how you have developed professionally through the course (knowledge, skills, values);
*   your learning needs as a preceptor in your first midwifery post.

Case study: Paul's development

The personal development I have achieved through the course

The course has meant a lot of learning for me. Learning alongside women and working with women and families from a different background from myself has been a rewarding and humbling experience. I think these are the important issues.

- *Being able now to listen much more openly to the meaning of women's experiences of their bodies and of childbirth.*
- *Being more open in my thinking – recognising that there are many ways of approaching an issue and it is important not to rush to judgement.*
- *Developing better skills in challenging – I think (hope) I am not so confrontational but instead more able to explore difference constructively.*

My professional development

I started the course with some professional experience, although I suspect I may have over-rated its relevance to midwifery and thinking about normal birth. Being a man on the course has been a challenge, and I have had to think carefully about responses to me (both positive and negative) and how these impact on my professional practice. The most significant learning has been:

- *really being able to grasp research and use it to guide my practice;*
- *appreciating the importance of reflection in developing critical thinking and academic learning;*
- *having a much deeper understanding of discrimination and its impact on people's lives;*
- *developing my interpersonal skills – understanding how other people may perceive me and knowing how to present myself in different situations – but still be me.*

My learning needs as a preceptor

I have been offered a post on the labour ward where I spent one placement, so my initial learning needs will mostly be related to my employment. I have identified them as:

- *enhancing my assessment and observation skills, particularly in situations where I might be distracted by external issues;*
- *developing my communication skills with other professionals – there will be lots of opportunities for this;*
- *keeping up my reading so I am able to inform my practice with up-to-date research;*
- *continuing to improve my skills in listening well to people – this links to developing a more empowering style of midwifery.*

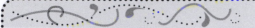

Chapter summary

This chapter has focused on learning at Level 6 of an undergraduate degree in midwifery. We have explored what it means to be an autonomous, independent learner and seen how it is relevant at this stage of your study. In particular, we have focused on metacognition, a facet of learning that can be promoted through reflection. The attributes of an independent, autonomous learner identified here will be required for the final stages of your study – on most courses this will involve writing a dissertation or completing another kind of independent project. We will explore this in more depth in Chapter 11. Implicit in this understanding of learning is that you will continue your professional development into and throughout your employment. By the end of your midwifery degree you should be ready to be a lifelong learner.

Further reading

Cottrell, S (2010) *Skills for success* (2nd edition). Basingstoke: Palgrave.

This very accessible book provides detailed advice about, and helpful activities for, personal development planning.

Cottrell, S (2013) *The study skills handbook* (4th edition). Basingstoke: Palgrave Macmillan.

This helpful book includes practical suggestions for managing your own study.

DH (2004) *The NHS Knowledge and Skills Framework (NHS KSF) and the Development Review Process*. London: DH.

NMC (2011) *The prep handbook*. London: NMC.

Chapter 11
Bringing your learning together
The dissertation

This chapter will help you to meet the Quality Assurance Agency for Higher Education (QAA, 2008) requirement that students studying at Level 6 are able to:

- demonstrate a systematic understanding of key aspects of their field of study, including acquisition of coherent and detailed knowledge, at least some of which is at, or informed by, the forefront of defined aspects of a discipline;
- apply the methods and techniques that they have learned to review, consolidate, extend and apply their knowledge and understanding and to initiate and carry out projects;
- critically evaluate arguments, assumptions, abstract concepts and data (that may be incomplete) to make judgements, and to frame appropriate questions to achieve a solution – or identify a range of solutions – to a problem;
- communicate information, ideas, problems and solutions to both specialist and non-specialist audiences.
- demonstrate the ability to manage their own learning and to make use of scholarly reviews and primary sources (for example, refereed research articles and/or original materials appropriate to the discipline).

NMC Standards for Pre-registration Midwifery Education

This chapter will address the following competencies:

Domain: Achieving quality care through evaluation and research

Apply relevant knowledge to the midwife's own practice in structured ways which are capable of evaluation. This will include:

- critical appraisal of knowledge and research evidence;
- critical appraisal of the midwife's own practice;
- gaining feedback from women and their families and appropriately applying this to practice;
- disseminating critically appraised good practice.

continued . . . •••

Inform and develop the midwife's own practice and the practice of others through using the best available evidence and reflecting on practice. This will include:

- keeping up to date with evidence;
- applying evidence to practice;
- alerting others to new evidence for them to apply to their own practice.

Chapter aims

After reading this chapter you will be able to:

- appreciate what is required in a dissertation;
- use planning, organisational and thinking skills to complete a project;
- synthesise a range of perspectives and knowledge about a topic to develop new thinking.

Introduction

In this chapter we will consider what is required of midwifery students at the final stage of their studies. While courses differ, on many these academic skills will be tested through an extended piece of written work, a project or a dissertation. The dissertation gives you the opportunity to:

- select your own topic and develop a particular interest;
- build on the foundation of your learning so far on the course;
- work, with the support of a tutor, in a self-directed and independent way;
- experience the process of producing knowledge;
- manage a project from beginning to end;
- demonstrate your academic assertiveness;
- consolidate your communication, information-seeking and intellectual skills;
- find your own voice, express your perspectives on a topic and hence make evident your professional development.

Within the constraints of course guidelines the dissertation can provide an opportunity for students to select their own topic, decide on their approach and work in a self-directed and independent way. It provides the opportunity for bringing together, using and extending learning on the course so far. Students who make the most of this find that their maturity as a learner is positively enhanced. This development equips them with skills and attributes that are directly transferable to employment and midwifery practice, such as the ability to work independently, time management, report writing, analysis and synthesis.

The dissertation

The dissertation differs significantly from other assessed work in length, depth and complexity. On some courses students may be expected to carry out small-scale original research, but this is not necessarily a requirement and will not be covered here. It is more likely that students will use research skills in searching for, and analysing, existing or secondary data. In the dissertation students have the opportunity to individually choose a topic of interest and, within the course assessment criteria, explore it in a way that fascinates them. It requires more prolonged, sustained and deeper engagement than standard essays and assignments.

Very little has been written about undergraduate dissertations, either generally or on midwifery courses. However, an internet search exploring course requirements suggests that in order to successfully complete their dissertations or projects, students will need to:

- select their own topic and find an appropriate focus;
- examine a relevant topic in depth;
- systematically search and review literature;
- select appropriate and relevant information;
- explore different perspectives on the topic;
- evaluate the material gathered;
- think critically, analytically and reflectively;
- manage the volume of material;
- organise their thinking;
- synthesise the range of perspectives and different knowledge on the topic;
- make relevant connections with the practice of midwifery;
- structure their work;
- use tutorial support;
- work independently and methodically;
- present a cogently argued, clearly written, logically structured piece of work.

Activity 11.1 — *Reflection*

The challenges of the dissertation

Reflect on yourself as a learner. What specific challenges does the dissertation present for you?

Comment

Later in the chapter we will explore some of these issues in more depth. Here it is worth remembering that in order to successfully complete your dissertation you will need to utilise, build on and develop further all the aspects of studying we have already considered.

- Making connections between theory, knowledge and practice (Chapters 3 and 6).
- Critical evaluation and analysis (Chapter 5).
- Being a reflective learner and practitioner (Chapter 7).
- Being research informed (Chapter 9).
- Being an independent autonomous learner (Chapter 10).

You may find it useful to revisit the chapters that are particularly relevant to the aspects of learning you find especially challenging.

Students' experiences

When thinking about working on your dissertation it may also be helpful to learn from other students who have successfully produced one.

Research summary: student views on dissertations

There is limited research on students' experience of completing undergraduate dissertations and integrated assignments. Below are some significant comments about how they found the process.

- The relative freedom to pursue your own topic was enjoyable.
- The sense of individual ownership of the work was motivating.
- Individual choice of the topic can lead to the study having real personal meaning.
- There was pleasure in mastering new ways of learning, seeing an issue from different perspectives, developing deeper understanding and managing the complexity of a big project.
- Working on the dissertation required high personal investment.
- It was very time consuming.
- Some students felt swamped by the size of the task.
- The experience was emotionally unsettling. (This appeared to be because students shifted between intellectual confusion and moments of insight and order.)
- Producing the dissertation was not easy but was worthwhile.
- General support from other students could be helpful, but because dissertations are so individual, talking to other students could be counterproductive and produce panic.
- Working constructively with a supervisor was very important.
- The final part was the most demanding but also the most rewarding.
- The submission date seemed almost artificial, as if it would never come, and then suddenly it arrived.
(Derounian, 2011; Todd et al., 2004; Watson et al., 2002)

These observations highlight that the dissertation requires great commitment and, because it involves developing new thinking, is demanding but also rewarding. Our experience suggests that part of the sense of achievement comes from rising to the demands and overcoming the challenges. Next we will explore three important learning approaches that should help you in this:

using supervision; organisation and planning; synthesis and problem solving. While these aspects of working on a dissertation have been separated out so they are clear for you, in practice you will find that they are closely related and can complement each other; for example, you can use your organisational skills to find ways of developing clarity about different approaches, and putting together an effective structure can be assisted by analytic and reflective thinking.

Using supervision

Most universities will allocate an individual supervisor for this piece of work. This can position you in a new and different learning relationship with a tutor. Previously it is likely that your tutorials will have been conducted in groups – now you will be working in a one-to-one academic relationship, possibly for the first time. Because of the importance of the dissertation and because this is an individual piece of work, it is likely to be a more intense process (Derounian, 2011; Hannigan and Burnard, 2001). You will be asked to present your thoughts and ideas and to share your work in progress. It is possible that you will feel exposed by this and anxious about appearing foolish. In our experience students sometimes unhelpfully avoid tutorials because of this fear. It is important to be reflective about your feelings about this tutorial relationship in order that you are able to use it as constructively as possible.

Tutors have a range of responsibilities while their students are working on dissertations. They may have subject expertise or they may be able to signpost you to other expert knowledge; they can help you decide on your topic and assist with formulating ideas; they will support you in managing the project through timetabling and organisation of resources; they can provide guidance on structuring and writing; they will read drafts and give you feedback; they will act as a mentor to aid your reflection and critical analytic thinking; they may provide editorial direction on your writing; they can advise you on issues of presentation including anonymisation.

Your responsibilities as a student include: attending all your tutorials; being punctual; arming yourself with questions and issues you want to raise and making sure you have read relevant material; being prepared to admit you do not understand if you are struggling with something; reading tutor feedback carefully; asking for clarification if you do not understand what your tutor has written or said; working hard between tutorials; keeping to agreed target dates. In short, your responsibility is to be an active and effective learner.

It is important to clarify with your tutor the practical boundaries of the tutorial, such as frequency, timing, cancellation, postponement and recording. You both need to be clear about your expectations of working together – for instance, what email or telephone contact is agreed as acceptable between tutorials. It is useful to record all these issues in an agreement. Derounian (2011, p98) provides a helpful example of such a contract. At the beginning of the work on your dissertation you may find you need more support as selecting a topic and finding an appropriate focus, together with planning targets for a piece of work of this size, are among the hardest aspects of the dissertation. As you proceed with the dissertation, learn how best to use feedback and become more confident, you should become a more autonomous learner and require less detailed guidance from your tutor (Todd et al., 2006). It can be helpful to keep a note of the meetings and other contacts with your tutor.

Activity 11.2 — Reflection

Using one-to-one tutorial support

Reflect on your feelings about one-to-one tutorial support. Identify the positives and negatives for you. Think about what you need to do to maximise the opportunity.

Case study: Linda and her dissertation tutor

Linda had submitted her dissertation topic as requested and had been allocated Martin Soames as her tutor. He had taught the Professional Midwifery for Practice module, and Linda had found him a little daunting. Other students thought she was lucky as he was perceived to be knowledgeable and challenging. However, Linda felt that under his scrutiny she would find it difficult to explain her ideas. Rather than arranging her first tutorial as was expected on the course timetable, she started working on her own. Over coffee Linda's critical friend Maggie enthused about her first tutorial – how it had been demanding but given her focus. Linda reluctantly shared with Maggie why she had not arranged to meet with Martin. Maggie helped her reflect on this, and Linda recalled experiences from school, and her nursing course, of feeling embarrassed when she did not get things right. Maggie encouraged her to get on with fixing a tutorial. Then Linda bumped into Martin in the corridor and he suggested a time. At the first tutorial Linda shared some of her anxieties with Martin. This was helpful in setting the context for their future work. Linda also quickly realised that if she had arranged the tutorial earlier, her initial work on the dissertation could have been more productive.

Organisation and planning

Being able to handle the size and complexity of the work involved in your dissertation is one aspect of becoming an autonomous learner. While you will have support from a tutor, the overall responsibility for managing the various aspects of the dissertation lies with you. Developing habits of self-motivation and self-discipline will help you to focus on the aspects set out below.

Select your topic and focus

As discussed above, this is a difficult stage. However, it should not be delayed, as time for working on your dissertation is at a premium. Remember that the dissertation is an opportunity to delve deeper and explore more about an aspect of midwifery that really gripped, puzzled or intrigued you.

When choosing your topic, you can focus your ideas by thinking about the following questions:

- Is it appropriate to midwifery?
- Does it engage you? Will it sustain your interest when your energy and enthusiasm are flagging?

- Is there sufficient, accessible and varied literature?
- Can you approach it analytically?
- Is it fit for assessment – will it enable you to meet the criteria required by the course?
- Is it too broad? It is normally better to aim for depth and quality rather than breadth. Students almost invariably begin with topics that are much too wide.

Within the topic you will then need to clarify your focus. Sometimes this can be done by formulating a question, which should be clear and straightforward. It might be framed in the form of a midwifery dilemma. This focus will set the boundaries for your dissertation and should be clear, contained and manageable. Unless you choose a narrow focus you risk producing a dissertation that is descriptive and general – and will therefore not meet the academic requirements at this level (Hannigan and Burnard, 2001).

Case study: Nazneen's dissertation

During Nazneen's third-year placement she became very interested in different aspects of cord clamping and proposed this as the topic for her dissertation. She had looked at some of the literature on the potential health benefits of 'delayed' cord clamping for babies, the relationship to the third stage of labour and how cord clamping might interfere with aspects of normal birth and bonding. At her first meeting with her tutor, Ellen, they agreed that there were many interesting aspects to the subject but that it would be more constructive to narrow her focus and decide which area she was really interested in. Ellen helped Nazneen to talk about some of her practice experiences with cord clamping and identified further, relevant literature.

By the end of the tutorial, Nazneen's overall topic had changed; she decided she wanted to explore how midwives can enhance the environment of care in the immediate period after birth. She would discuss cord clamping in one chapter but the main focus would be the midwife's role in nurturing the new family and how decisions made about cord clamping could impact on the birth experience for the mother and the baby. She was still very interested in the issue of cord clamping and resuscitation, particularly in pre-term babies, but now realised she was more interested in the midwives' role at this significant time for mothers and babies and families.

Setting and using a timetable

Effective time management is fundamental to thorough work on your dissertation and its successful completion. It is helpful to set out a clear timetable of work, with targets. Working backwards from the deadline, you should aim to complete all stages a week before the submission date. This makes allowance for the inevitable crises: not being able to access literature; the computer blowing up; family problems; illness; and any other unexpected demands. Your timetable should link to the structure and can help you to work out what needs to be done first, the different stages of the dissertation and planning ahead. Allowing yourself time to revise early drafts and to read the dissertation as a whole can avoid unnecessary repetition and ensure connections are made between different sections.

You will need to plan how to make time for working on your dissertation as there may be other demands on your time such as practice placements. So you need to figure out how best to use the time available – for instance, when it is most helpful for you to take breaks and how to use them constructively to re-energise yourself. Understanding which, for you, are the most productive times of the day and maximising these can be balanced with finding easier tasks to do when you are tired or less able to take on challenging tasks.

The literature search and reading

You will be expected to be aware of up-to-date research, literature, legislation and policies and guidance, which will probably mean that journals and other electronic information are more relevant and helpful to you than textbooks. The pace of knowledge development is now so rapid that many textbooks are out of date before they are printed. Your main sources of research are those outlined in Chapter 8, page 120, but be prepared to search historical sources that may not be as readily available electronically.

Beware of time-wasting searches – your tutor or librarian should be able to give you guidance on using search terms for your subject to avoid fruitless activity. Always read the abstracts of journal articles and reviews with your topic in mind so that you can be clear about their potential usefulness.

Aim to read in a purposeful and focused way, bearing in mind the themes in your dissertation but without being too blinkered. As you read, you should be alert to how different theories, aspects of research and knowledge, perspectives and values relate to the focus of your dissertation and to each other. How well do they explain the issue? Do they build on each other? Are they complementary or contradictory? Keep clear notes and use highlighting and sticky notes to mark significant points or passages.

Using organisational skills

One practical way of managing the complexity of the dissertation is to make sure your organisational skills are good. You need a system of keeping papers, books, notes and drafts where you can easily find them. When you start you will probably not foresee how much material you will generate. Write everything down – your thoughts, struggles, lists of resources you need and issues you need to pursue – a notebook or tablet/iPad can be useful for this. Ensure you systematically keep a note of the references you are using from the beginning. It is most frustrating to have to search for a piece of information, such as the date of publication, when your time could be better used editing and improving your work. Software that assists the organisation of referencing may be helpful. You will also need to have a means of organising your thoughts, especially as the complexity of the topic develops and you explore different perspectives. Mind maps or colour coding can help to manage this material.

Finally, you need a good overall draft structure for the dissertation before you start writing. This usually necessitates identifying the main themes, each of which will be covered in a chapter. In addition, each chapter should be structured before you begin to write. Draft structures can always be revised in the light of new theories, research or insights. However, without this level of organisation, you can easily lose focus and spend unproductive time. Having examples of dissertations written by students in previous years can assist you in appreciating how good organisation and structure can help you meet the requirements of your course.

Case study: Paul's dissertation structure

Paul chose to write his dissertation on 'Non-pharmacological approaches to pain relief in labour'. This decision arose from his observations of home birth and reading on comfort and pain relief early in the course (see Chapter 3). He had later read a research review that revealed the lack of research into non-pharmacological forms of pain relief or comfort in labour (see Chapter 8). These thoughts and experiences motivated him to develop his understanding further. His tutor, Kate, helped him to organise the preliminary structure as shown below.

Chapter 1: Introduction

- *The topic and my focus; why I chose the topic.*
- *My observations of approaches to pain relief on placements.*
- *The questions I want to explore.*
- *How I went about searching for relevant material; the rationale for my choices; gaps in the literature.*
- *The structure and organisation of the dissertation.*

Chapter 2: Theories about pain

- *An exploration of theories about pain and its relief from medicine, psychology and sociology with specific reference to childbirth; summary and evaluation of the contribution of each theory.*

Chapter 3: Evidence from research

- *An outline of research studies and reviews on non-pharmacological approaches to pain relief in childbirth (covering acupuncture, massage, reflexology, aromatherapy, sterile water injections, TENS, relaxation and massage); a summary of the findings of the research and their implications for midwifery practice; limitations of the research.*

Chapter 4: Evidence from other sources

- *Historical accounts of pain and pain relief in childbirth; the views of midwives.*
- *Accounts from women and their partners; reflection on my practice experiences.*
- *A summary of the main themes, noting similarities and differences.*
- *Brief discussion of professional issues in relation to appropriate training and competency to administer therapies and medication.*

Chapter 5: Discussion of all the findings

- *The relative contributions of theories, research and experiences; how they relate to current policy; a synthesis of the evidence.*

Chapter 6: Conclusion and recommendations

- *Having explored this issue in depth, what are my conclusions?*
- *Recommendations for future practice.*

References and bibliography

Appendices

Activity 11.3   *Decision making*

Developing a structure

Read in detail the assessment criteria for the dissertation, project or extended essay on your course. Then, with a topic in mind, put together a structure that will provide a framework within which you can organise your study.

Writing and editing

Aim to write clearly and concisely, remembering your audience. Go back through the feedback you have received from previous assignments to identify your strengths and weaknesses in writing, and actively take steps to improve in the ways suggested. As you write, check that your arguments are clear and logical from sentence to sentence, from paragraph to paragraph and from chapter to chapter. After you have completed your first draft, read through it for different purposes – for sense, for clarity of your arguments, for typographical errors, for correct punctuation and grammar and for appropriate referencing. This will mean reading it many times – but without this you may not be able to proofread with the thoroughness required. If you have a friend who knows nothing about the subject, particularly if English is not their first language, asking them to read it can give you a valuable indicator of the clarity of your writing. Ensure you have met the assessment criteria and word length requirements for your course.

The skills outlined above are necessary for successful completion of your dissertation, but they are not sufficient. In the next section we will explore the academic skills needed.

Synthesis and identifying new thinking

Here we look at managing complexity, with specific attention to meeting the requirements of the dissertation. Complexity arises from the sheer number of sources of knowledge you might draw on, the different kinds of knowledge, constructed in varying ways, and the diverse perspectives that you will be confronted with. Here we will focus on how to deal with these different contributions to understanding a topic in midwifery and consider how they can be brought together, or synthesised, in order to be able to appreciate and understand an issue in a new way.

To synthesise means to combine different elements into a coherent whole. For example, in music a synthesiser generates and combines signals of different frequencies to make new sounds. At Level 6 of your studies you are expected to be able to synthesise the different, and often competing, views on an issue; achieving this successfully can lead to identifying new ways of understanding or perceiving an issue and the implications for midwifery policy and practice. Next we consider some stages in this process of learning – achieving synthesis and identifying new directions. In order to manage practically the volume of material you will assemble for your dissertation, it can be helpful to follow these stages for each of the chapters.

Drawing on different sources of knowledge

The possible ways of understanding any topic in midwifery, and hence what you would need to include in your dissertation, might be drawn from:

- theories that aim to explain the issue;
- midwifery values and ethics;
- research studies and reviews;
- midwifery practitioner knowledge and experience or practice wisdom;
- knowledge from the experiences of different groups of people who use maternity services;
- knowledge from the experience of families.

In each of these areas – particularly, theories, research and values – you are likely to find more than you can possibly include in your dissertation. Hence you need to be selective, choosing those theories that you consider best throw light on the topic and research studies that are most helpful in developing understanding. You must be clear about your reasons for this selection and justify your decision within the dissertation. When making your selection it is important to think about the different levels at which midwifery can be understood: the societal and structural level; the organisational level of policy and procedures; and the level of day-to-day practice. Aim to use theories and research concerned with each level. This enables you to take a holistic approach to the topic, showing that you grasp the significance of understanding the individual and day-to-day practice in a wider structural context of inequality and disadvantage.

Contested and competing knowledge

Of the theories and research you select, each can provide a lens for viewing the question or issue, presenting you with a new angle on the topic. Every perspective you include will impart a different understanding, telling a distinct story about a situation. You need to ensure you have a clear understanding of all the theories, research, values and perspectives you select, in order that you can work with them at a higher academic level. If you are struggling with a particular theory, you could discuss it with your tutor. You may find it helpful to refer back to Chapter 3, where some guidelines for grasping theory were set out, or to Chapter 8, in which we explored some ways of understanding research.

Evaluation, critical analysis and reflection

Once you have achieved clarity you should critically analyse, reflect on and evaluate each of the areas on knowledge and understanding on which you are drawing. Using evaluation and critical analysis, as explored in Chapters 4, 5 and 9, will enable you to identify:

- the strengths and weakness of the diverse theories, research, knowledge and perspectives you have selected;
- the relevance and contribution of each to understanding of the topic;
- the consistency of each with the values of midwifery.

Taking a reflective approach, as outlined in Chapters 7 and 10, should ensure you understand why you might be more drawn to some theories and perspectives than others, and the implications of this for your analysis and evaluation.

Relating the ideas to each other

Consider the relative strengths and weaknesses of each of your sources in relation to each other

Considering sources of knowledge in relation to each other is a step towards managing the complexity of different understandings. For instance, you might find that accounts from women are strong on conveying feelings and building a picture of what it is like to be a recipient of services but relatively weak on theorising explanations for services being organised in particular ways. In contrast, a research study might have identified ten different models for organising services but might not cover the impact of each on the recipients of the service.

Consider the relative merits of the sources in relation to each other

Considering the different sources of knowledge in relation to each other means asking whether they reinforce, support, contradict or challenge each other – or whether they are linked in other ways. Aim to appreciate their differences and commonalities. If you have carried out your reading in a focused way, alert to the need for this kind of analysis, you will find it easier to achieve the necessary clarity.

Hold these competing ideas simultaneously

Aim to hold in your mind, simultaneously and in creative tension, the different perspectives, without drawing conclusions or rushing to judgement. This is complex and may be assisted by using diagrams and coloured marker pens to graphically illustrate differences and connections.

Make connections and develop arguments

Finally, make relevant connections between the ideas you have generated that throw light on the midwifery topic you have chosen. Develop arguments that incorporate and explain these ideas. In this way you should be able to build an integrated and cohesive account relating to the focus of your topic – answering the question or providing an explanation for the dilemma you originally posed. Aiming to put these ideas in writing clearly can alert you to aspects of your thinking that are not yet fully worked through. This may require you to retrace your steps and re-examine and rework your ideas.

Use this understanding to develop new thinking

Once you have explored the topic thoroughly and thrown new light on it, your insights should lead to new and innovative thinking. This might mean a different approach to practice, a changed understanding of an aspect of midwifery, the possible resolution of a practice dilemma or a proposed different direction for policy. Sometimes students are so relieved to have completed the other parts of the dissertation that they do not give sufficient attention to this final part. It can be helpful to ensure that this aspect of your dissertation is included in your structure from the beginning so you ensure it is not neglected or squeezed out.

Activity 11.4   *Critical thinking*

Synthesising your material

Think about one chapter or theme within your dissertation and follow the steps above to achieve synthesis of your material and the development of new thinking.

Case study: Nazneen's dissertation

Within the constraints of this book it is difficult to provide an in-depth, detailed and fully worked instance of synthesis and developing new thinking as required in a dissertation. However, the small-scale example presented below should provide an illustration.

The interim dissertation title that Nazneen agreed with her tutor Ellen was 'Nurturing the transition to family life in an undisturbed environment of care'. This was a working title that might change, but one that Nazneen and Ellen thought would help her to focus on the key elements of the dissertation: normal birth, promoting breastfeeding and protecting the new mother and baby from unwarranted interference in this very important time.

The focus of one chapter was the impact of later cord clamping. Nazneen thought she would need to include some context to the issue of cord clamping, but was aware from her discussions with Ellen that she needed to retain the main focus and not drift too far into discussion of other themes. This is a summary of Nazneen's notes and work in progress.

Drawing on different sources of knowledge

Below are the sources I drew on, organised by theme, with a précis of their relevance.

Physical benefits of later cord clamping

McDonald, S and Middleton, P *(2008) Effect of timing of umbilical cord clamping of term infants on maternal and neonatal outcomes.* Cochrane Database of Systematic-reviews *Issue 3.*

This review of 11 trials concludes that delayed clamping of the cord does not appear to increase the risk of post-partum haemorrhage. It discusses the problems of definitions of 'delayed' and notes that late cord clamping improves the iron status for babies without increasing risks of post-partum haemorrhage. The risk of jaundice requiring phototherapy in delayed cord clamping is also considered.

Gabriel, M A M, Martin, I L, Escobar, A L et al. *(2010) Randomized controlled trial of early skin-to-skin contact: effects on the mother and the newborn.* Acta Paediatrica, *99 (11): 1630–34.*

This small study found that skin-to-skin care promoted thermo-regulation in the newborn and an increase in exclusive breastfeeding at hospital discharge.

Mercer, J and Erikson-Owens, D *(2010) Evidence for neonatal transition and the first hour of life. In Walsh, D and Downe, S (eds)* Intrapartum care *(Essential Midwifery Practice). Oxford: Wiley-Blackwell, pp81–93.*

The authors note that immediate cord clamping reduces neonatal blood volume by 25–50 per cent, and limiting this supply to the baby potentially interferes with optimal neonatal transition. In contrast, later cord clamping can both prevent iron deficiency and blood loss and ensure that babies receive their full allotment of stem cells at birth. The physical and psychological advantages of later cord clamping are also discussed in depth.

Emotional/psychological considerations

Fahy, K, Hastie, C, Bisits, A et al. *(2010) Holistic physiological care compared with active management of the third stage of labour for woman at low risk of postpartum haemorrhage: a cohort study.* Women and birth, *23 (4): 146–52.*

This is a study in Australia that concluded that 'holistic psychophysiological' care in the third stage of labour is safe for women with low risk of post-partum haemorrhage. This approach supports the integration of the woman's mind, spirit and body, and it is argued that it provides benefits for both mother and baby.

Odent, M *(2008) Birth territory: the besieged territory for the obstetrician. In Fahy, K, Foureur, M and Hastie, C (eds)* Birth territory and midwifery guardianship: theory for practice, education and research. *Edinburgh: Books for Midwives, pp131–48.*

Odent identifies the important needs in childbirth – safety, privacy and warmth – and emphasises the strong connection between safety and privacy in an undisturbed environment of care. He argues that distraction in the third stage could increase fight or flight hormone levels and indirectly increase the risk of bleeding.

Walsh, D *(2010) Birth environment. In Walsh, D and Downe, S (eds)* Intrapartum care *(Essential Midwifery Practice). Oxford: Wiley-Blackwell, pp45–62.*

In this chapter Denis Walsh argues that women seek social and psychological safety in the birth environment and that practice should provide compassion, warmth, comfort and protection. He cites one theory that suggests that the physical act of cord clamping interrupts this.

National guidelines on cord clamping

NICE (National Institute of Clinical [Care] Excellence) *(2007)* CG55: Intrapartum care. *London: NICE.*

NICE currently recommends a managed third stage with immediate cord clamping. The guidelines do, however, recommend keeping mother and baby undisturbed for up to an hour particularly in relation to the promotion of breastfeeding

Mothers' views on birth

Green, J M and Baston, G A *(2003) Feeling in control during labour: concepts, correlates and consequences.* Birth, *30 (4): 235–47.*

This study highlights the importance of the birth environment in providing security and control for women. They also link dissatisfaction with the birth experience and lack of involvement in decisions to a higher incidence of postnatal depression.

continued . . .

Cultural aspects

In one of my discussion groups there was a lively debate about skin-to-skin contact. Some students had observed that a peaceful and close time for mothers and babies immediately after the birth had been wonderful for them and that fathers had found it pleasurable to be part of that experience. Breastfeeding seemed to follow on comfortably. However, some women seemed to want to hold their baby after the baby had been wiped and wrapped and were uncomfortable with the idea of skin-to-skin contact. Various theories were put forward within the group – for example, that some women find the thought of blood and fluids of birth to be unpleasant or frightening. Some stereotypical views were expressed about particular groups of women while others argued that an individual approach should be taken with each woman.

Forde, P *(1999) Sensitive midwifery.* Midwifery Today-International Midwife, *49, 60–61.*

This article advocates that midwives should learn to be sensitive and listen for those silent messages that the women and their families communicate.

Cortis, J D *(2000) Multi-culturalism and what else?* Nurse Education Today, *20: 65–67.*

Cortis argues that, while it may be useful to have background knowledge about a cultural group, it would be dangerous to assume that all members of the group adhere to all the observable norms of that cultural group, as this may lead to stereotyping of people in terms of their cultures, races and faiths.

Practitioner issues

Farrar, D, Tuffnell, D, Airey, R and Duley, L *(2010) Care during the third stage of labour: a postal survey of UK midwives and obstetricians.* BMC Pregnancy and Childbirth, *10.1186/1471–2393–10–23.*

The authors question the confidence of practitioners in relation to cord clamping and changing practice in third stage. One study shows that 93 per cent of obstetricians and 73 per cent of midwives always, or usually, use active management with a variety of techniques.

Seibo, C, Licqurish, S and Rolls, C *(2010) 'Lending the space': midwives' perceptions of birth space and clinical risk management.* Midwifery, *265: 526–31.*

The authors suggest that midwives' concerns regarding risk and compliance with guidelines may inhibit their confidence in decision making and planning care, the promotion of normal birth and the effectiveness of interventions.

Evaluation, critical analysis and reflection

These are the some of the points I considered:

- *The research and material on which I have drawn are from reputable academic sources that have been subject to peer review or editorial scrutiny – apart from our group reflection on experience which had a different value.*
- *The research suggests benefits of later cord clamping for mothers and babies.*

continued . . .

- *Studies on the third stage of labour are unclear about which elements of a managed third stage are crucial to reducing the risk of blood loss.*
- *I found it very interesting to note, in some of the literature, a separation between physical and emotional aspects.*
- *There is a continuing debate about cord clamping within the context of third-stage management.*
- *There seems to be a lack of research on mothers' experiences and views on cord clamping, but it seems appropriate to generalise from other literature about women's views on control and choices in labour and birth.*
- *In practice I have seen a variety of techniques. Later cord clamping was often linked to a quieter and nurturing environment while earlier cord clamping was more likely to be a noisier experience with the speedy processing of midwifery jobs taking precedence. In general, women appear to accept the approach taken by the midwife. I wonder how this relates to women-centred practice.*

Relating the ideas to each other

From my reading there is growing evidence of the physical and psychological benefits of later cord clamping. There is variation in current practice. It is apparent from the literature that women need midwives to be sensitive to their individual preferences and cultural needs, and this has relevance for decisions about cord clamping. NICE guidelines in relation to cord clamping have not yet changed, and this contributes to the uncertainties that midwives may feel about changing practice.

New thinking

- *Decisions about cord clamping are crucial to the experience of mothers and babies in the significant period post birth.*
- *In addition to the physiological benefits or otherwise of later cord clamping, the emotional impact on the mother and the baby needs to be integrated into thinking and research.*
- *Cord clamping is not a single intervention that can be looked at in isolation.*
- *There is a need for focused research on third-stage interventions and the impact on the transition to family life. Cord clamping is one element of this.*
- *As practice changes, outcomes need to be carefully monitored for unanticipated effects, both positive and negative.*
- *Midwives need the confidence to weigh up the impact for new families of intervention at the time of birth, focusing on the overall picture of health and well-being.*

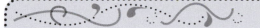

Chapter summary

In this chapter we have explored the dissertation, which for many of you will be the final, and most demanding, piece of work of your degree. While it has not been possible to consider every aspect in detail, the focus here has aimed to help you understand the purpose and requirements of a dissertation and to provide you with ways of going about such a project. Ultimately, most students seem to appreciate having the opportunity to challenge themselves and produce such an individual piece of work. We hope you do too.

Further reading

Aveyard, H (2010) *Doing a literature review in health and social care* (2nd edition). Buckingham: Open University Press.

Hart, C (1998) *Doing a literature review: releasing the social science research imagination.* London: Sage.

Both these books are useful guides to carrying out a literature review.

There are several websites that provide advice on dissertations. Many of these are focused on higher, not undergraduate, degrees and therefore may be misleading – so use with caution.

Cottrell, S (2013) *The study skills handbook* (4th edition). Basingstoke: Palgrave Macmillan.

This book includes a dissertation checklist and action plan that may be useful in helping you with organisation.

Whittaker, A and Williamson, G R (2011) *Succeeding in research project plans and literature reviews for nursing students.* London: Sage/Learning Matters.

Written for nursing students, this book focuses on the final year extended piece of work

Chapter 12
Dealing with complexity
Using knowledge in practice

This chapter will help you to meet the Quality Assurance Agency for Higher Education (QAA, 2008) requirement that students studying at Level 6 are able to:

- demonstrate conceptual understanding that enables the student:
  - to devise and sustain arguments and/or to solve problems using ideas and techniques, some of which are at the forefront of a discipline;
  - to describe and comment upon particular aspects of current research, or equivalent advanced scholarship, in the discipline;
- demonstrate an appreciation of the uncertainty, ambiguity and limits of knowledge;
- critically evaluate arguments, assumptions, abstract concepts and data (that may be incomplete) to make judgements, and to frame appropriate questions to achieve a solution – or identify a range of solutions – to a problem;
- communicate information, ideas, problems and solutions to both specialist and non-specialist audiences.

NMC Standards for Pre-registration Midwifery Education

This chapter will address the following competencies:

Domain: Professional and ethical practice
Practise in accordance with relevant legislation. This will include:

- demonstrating knowledge of contemporary ethical issues and their impact on midwifery practice;
- managing the complexities arising from ethical and legal dilemmas.

Domain: Developing the individual midwife and others
Review, develop and enhance the midwife's own knowledge, skills and fitness to practise. This will include:

- reflecting on the midwife's own practice and making the necessary changes as a result.

continued . . .

Domain: Achieving quality care through evaluation and research

Apply relevant knowledge to the midwife's own practice in structured ways which are capable of evaluation. This will include:

- critical appraisal of knowledge and research evidence;
- critical appraisal of the midwife's own practice;
- disseminating critically appraised good practice.

Inform and develop the midwife's own practice and the practice of others through using the best available evidence and reflecting on practice. This will include:

- keeping up to date with evidence;
- applying evidence to practice.

Chapter aims

After reading this chapter you will be able to:

- appreciate the reasons for the complexity of midwifery practice;
- identify some skills and strategies for working within complexity.

Introduction

One factor in the decision that midwifery should become a graduate profession was the recognition that sophisticated academic skills are needed for competent practice. This was acknowledgement of the complexity of current midwifery practice in which critical, analytical and reflective ability is required to practise with confidence. In this chapter we will discuss some aspects of this complexity before considering strategies for using higher-level academic skills constructively to support positive ways of working in this environment.

The complex nature of midwifery

We will begin by considering in more detail the nature of current midwifery practice, focusing on three aspects: the context of practice; ethical dilemmas; and the many sources of knowledge in midwifery. At this stage of your course you should have a sound awareness of such issues, from both your studies and your placements. Our discussion here will build on the themes covered in earlier chapters – the aim is to help you to make better sense of your experiences.

The context of practice

There is now robust evidence that midwifery care is safe and cost-effective (Schroeder et al., 2012). There is an increased interest in midwife-led births from government and national organisations (RCOG, 2011), and midwives continue to be positive about supporting home birth (RCM, 2011a) but midwives and their leaders have voiced concerns about the future of maternity services.

Professor Lesley Page, the president of the Royal College of Midwives, observes from her visits to maternity services all over the UK:

> *In general there are too few midwives, current services are usually overstretched, work beyond capacity and are under great pressure . . . [with staff] . . . working hard to maintain safe, high quality services . . . leading development in new approaches to care, transforming practice and developing new services . . . [Midwives demonstrate] . . . courageous and painstaking commitment and work, often against a background of resistance to change.*
> (Page, 2013, p6)

Paul Lewis (2013, p158) concurs:

> *too many women in the UK are experiencing maternity care that does not respect their basic rights. [There is] strain on under-resourced maternity services, a culture of excessive emphasis on clinical policy rather than individualised care.*

In a more general context, Schön (1983, p42) writes graphically of professional practice as *the swampy lowland where situations are confusing 'messes'*. He also asserts that this is where the greatest problems of human concern for practitioners occur.

In order to develop constructive ways of working in the current, challenging context, it can be helpful first to develop an analysis of the reasons for this.

Activity 12.1   *Reflection*

Understanding the context of midwifery practice analytically

Identify some explanations for the state of current midwifery practice. Then compare your analysis with the analysis set out below.

Considerable organisational change

In April 2013 the structure and organisation of the NHS changed significantly. It is now overseen nationally by the NHS Commissioning Board. Locally, clinical commissioning boards made up of GPs will purchase services (Campbell, 2012). The implications of this for health services generally and for maternity services locally are not yet clear. However, such change inevitably engenders anxiety and uncertainty about the funding of services, the criteria by which decisions will be made about allocation of contracts and the type of services that will be given priority.

The constraints imposed by resource limitations

McInnes and McIntosh (2012) argue that public sector cuts across the UK give cause for concern in maternity services. They cite evidence – provided by the media, academic sources and professional bodies – of inadequately staffed services. In particular, a report from the Royal College of Midwives (RCM, 2011b) noted high and increasing birth rates in all four UK countries. The 'baby boom' in England and Wales, compounded by understaffing, has led to a chronic shortage of midwives.

Factors that contribute towards pregnancy and childbirth becoming more complex

Particular factors related to societal changes have contributed to pregnancy and childbirth becoming more complex. The childbearing population is generally older and presents more complex pregnancies in general, together with additional complications related to assisted conception (RCM, 2011b). There is a higher rate of multiple births; more women survive serious childhood illness, become pregnant and need extra care; there is increasing social and ethnic diversity, sometimes leading to communication difficulties and other social and clinical challenges in maternity care (Chief Nursing Officers of England, Northern Ireland, Scotland and Wales, 2010). At the same time the changing clinical profile of childbearing women indicates poorer general health due to unhealthy lifestyle factors such as smoking, alcohol misuse, use of recreational drugs, poor diet (CEMACE, 2011) and increasing obesity. Obesity is associated with poorer outcomes in pregnancy and clinical complications such as heart disease and diabetes. These factors create greater complexity in pregnancy and childbirth, and provide challenges to the provision of maternity care and to the workloads of midwives.

Working in a context that is not always conducive to creative and woman-centred practice

Kirkham (2013) notes the different, but co-existing, models of midwifery – the medical and the industrial – and contrasts these with the optimal circumstances for pregnancy and birth, which should create a feeling of safety and trust. The medical model, she argues, has been prevalent in maternity care. Its hierarchical approach holds doctors as the experts with greatest control over the patient. It tends to lead towards thinking in opposites – where one extreme is seen as good/normal (breast/home) and the other bad/abnormal (bottle/hospital). Such 'one size fits all' thinking prevents consideration of what might be possible between these artificially created extremes and can create fear of difference and performance anxiety. The aim of the industrial model is efficient throughput leading to centralisation into large hospitals; there is pressure to conform and standardise through protocols, guidelines and polices. Although women are described as consumers who can exercise choice, this choice is restricted by centralisation and standardisation. This model, too, creates fears and constrains the potential for developing innovative, women-centred practice.

Jowitt (2013) highlights the growth of a 'control and command' culture in the NHS and regrets its impact on midwifery. However, she also notes the hope for a different approach contained in the *Report of the Mid Staffordshire NHS Foundation Trust Public Inquiry* (Francis, 2013), which asserted the need for a focus on the individual experiences that lie behind statistics, benchmarks and action plans.

These factors combine to create a context for practice that will by now undoubtedly be familiar to you.

Activity 12.2 *Reflection*

Examples from your placement

For each of the explanations given for the challenging nature of current midwifery practice, identify an example from your placement.

Ethical dilemmas in midwifery practice

We first explored values in Chapter 2, considering their fundamental importance to midwifery practice and noting the role of the shared set of values set out in *Midwives rules and standards* (NMC, 2012). Students and midwives can find that integrating values into their work is not straightforward, and they are often posed with ethical dilemmas. In such situations midwives are faced with two or more apparently contradictory values; they need to be able to find a way forward that takes both into account. For example, they may be faced with balancing the following values.

- A woman's right to choice *with* potential risk to herself or her baby.
- Respecting confidentiality *with* sharing information with colleagues and other agencies.
- A midwife's personal values *with* midwifery values.
- Obligations to women and their families *with* accountability to employers.

Activity 12.3 *Decision making*

Identifying an ethical dilemma

Identify an ethical dilemma that you have come across in practice. Write down the competing values that you found you were trying to resolve.

Case study: Nazneen's dilemma about Francesca

Nazneen and her mentor Paula are having a difficult shift supporting Francesca, who has arrived at the main obstetric unit in strong labour. They have learnt that Francesca is 38 years old and having her second child. She has a 14-year-old daughter, is divorced and runs her own restaurant. Nazneen is surprised that Francesca has no hand-held notes and then even more startled to learn that she has concealed her pregnancy from everyone she

continued . . .

> knows, having told her family she is staying overnight with friends in London. Francesca refuses to talk about the father of the baby but says that she is '39 weeks exactly' and that she does not wish to see or touch the baby. Her plan is go straight home after the birth and 'not look back'. Nazneen and Paula try to prepare Francesca for the rapidly approaching birth while also attempting to confirm gestation and other key factors in her medical and obstetric history, without notes and against a background of no antenatal care. Francesca's blood pressure is very high on a first and subsequent reading, and Nazneen and Paula need to tell Francesca at some point that she will need to stay in hospital after the birth so that her blood pressure can be safely monitored. Although she is very busy dealing with the practical aspects of the birth, Nazneen is also aware of the competing values in this situation, which she has identified as:
>
> Francesca's right to choice and self-determination versus the potential risks to her health and to the welfare of her baby.

Midwifery knowledge derives from multiple sources

The third related factor contributing to the complexity of midwifery concerns the multiple sources of the knowledge upon which decision making in practice is based. Gimenez's (2012) research into undergraduate writing in a UK university suggests that midwifery is seen as both a science and an art. From science it uses clinical knowledge, incorporating logical reasoning and empirical data such as the anatomy and physiology of mother and baby, and clinical competence (including reflective practice). From art it draws on intuitive and embodied knowledge, gained from personal experience and professional observation, together with thinking about the wider context of midwifery. The midwifery students in Gimenez's study identified that they found it difficult to reconcile the science and art of midwifery and wondered where one finished and the other started. Another problem they identified was the combining of different sources of evidence, noting that sometimes the sources could clash and even be contradictory.

Working in and with complexity

In the next section of the chapter we will identify some ways of thinking and practising in the complexity outlined in the first section. All of these approaches build on academic skills already covered in the book – skills in evaluation, analysis, reflection and **critical thinking**. Without these abilities you will find it difficult to make progress and successfully study at Level 6 of the midwifery degree. If you find yourself struggling, you may find it useful to revisit earlier chapters.

Aim to be 'knowing' and 'not knowing'

The complexity and uncertainty of midwifery has been explored above. Because there is a tendency to want the comfort of certainty, working in this context can be anxiety provoking. One response to this unease can be unhelpful, concrete thinking that may mean neglecting to consider an issue from different perspectives using a range of knowledge and competing theoretical explanations. Ainsworth (2013, p9) argues that taking a position of 'knowing' is limiting. She argues that midwives can be more engaging and creative when they consciously choose a position of both 'knowing' and 'not knowing', which provides the potential for finding a 'new way', as yet maybe not conceived.

It is therefore important for students and midwives to develop the capacity to live with not knowing – appreciating that there may not be one correct answer, and actively seeking out and embracing other knowledge and versions of the truth. In this way, complexity of understanding can be developed. This can have real practice significance, as it can help avoid inappropriate certainty about the judgement of situations. However, this approach also means learning to manage the anxiety generated by not having a clear solution, developing the ability to live with doubt and uncertainty while taking the time to seek other accounts. For some midwives, practising in this way may be anxiety provoking. Managing such powerful emotions will be assisted by self-reflection and the constructive use of supervision.

Activity 12.4   *Reflection*

Working in uncertainty

Think about your ability to work in *secure unknowingness*. Reflect on how you respond to lack of certainty and the impact on your practice.

Case study: Paul assists with Teresa's labour and birth

Paul and Kelly, his mentor, are attending the home birth of Teresa and Mark's third baby. All has been straightforward, and the labour is progressing well. Teresa has a history of depression but found that having her second baby at home really helped her cope with the birth and the first few weeks after childbirth. She is therefore very keen to repeat this experience. This will be Paul's '40th baby' and he is thrilled that it will be another home birth.

There are signs that Teresa might be nearing second stage, and a 'show' is evident on the sheets and waterproof mats. Paul and Kelly make a note of the amounts initially, and then again when it seems to increase and involve some frank red loss. They know they must make a decision about whether to prepare for transfer to hospital. Although Teresa could have the baby at any moment, they are also aware that sometimes third labours are less predictable in terms of rapid progress. The blood loss may increase and herald problems for the labour and birth. Or it may, in retrospect, turn out to be a generous show that can precede a rapid second stage with a normal outcome in terms of blood loss. Paul and Kelly try to gently introduce the idea of transferring to hospital.

Teresa is very upset and emotional and says: 'I'll just lock myself in the bathroom and refuse to go if you call an ambulance.' Mark is shell-shocked and silent, and disappears from the room on the pretext of seeing to the other children.

In this situation of many unpredictable factors, Paul and Kelly need to manage any anxiety they feel, convey calm, confidence and clarity to Teresa, prepare for different outcomes and, drawing on their knowledge and

continued . . .

experience, plan for the safety of both the mother and the baby. They make a realistic plan for transfer to hospital but are also prepared for the possibility of a rapid birth and a post-partum haemorrhage and even for resuscitation of the baby.

Initially, Teresa appears to be inconsolable but is reassured that the ambulance and paramedics have been called to be on standby – not automatically for transfer to hospital, but rather to be ready should their skills and equipment be needed. Paul carefully and calmly outlines the possibilities and finds he is able to describe the potential scenarios in a realistic way that does not frighten Teresa. Kelly gives very positive feedback to Paul afterwards and helps him reflect on how they conveyed professional confidence and competence to Teresa and Mark in a challenging situation of unpredictable possibilities.

Use your thinking skills to resolve ethical dilemmas

Working within the complexity of midwifery you will find you need to find resolutions to ethical dilemmas. This can be a difficult balancing act; using the following steps may help you to use your analytic and creative thinking skills.

- *Spell out the competing values and think about the principles behind them.* It can be helpful to clearly set these out.
- *Articulate the implications of different courses of action.* Use your analytic thinking to identify the implications of the different courses of action implicit in each value position.
- *Keep the significance of working with women as a guiding principle.* Never lose sight of the importance of the value of practice that is in partnership with the labouring woman.
- *Build on your developing knowledge and experience to make professional judgement.* As your midwifery career progresses, you will be more able to judge whether learning from another situation can be helpfully deployed in new circumstances. Eraut (1994) argues that it is this interpretation of and application of learning and experience that constitutes professional judgement. Such expertise involves innovation and artistry as well as critical and analytic thinking, and midwives also need to use creativity in resolving dilemmas and finding ways forward.
- *Knowing why you have chosen a particular course of action.* You should be able to articulate your chosen course of action and justify it, clearly spelling out your reasons.

Case study: Nazneen explains her dilemma about Francesca

I needed to think carefully about the values and principles that guided my work. I knew that I needed to be 'with' Francesca in order to support her through the birth, but this was difficult because Francesca had not accessed ante-natal care and intended to leave after the birth. Francesca seemed so fixed and determined to go ahead with this, yet I was very aware of my responsibility for Francesca's after-care and for the welfare of the unborn baby. I found it hard to understand that a woman would not want to see and hold her baby. I found it hard to imagine why this would be the case. It was beyond my experience. Despite all this I wanted to find the best way forward and took the opportunity to talk it though with Paula. Together we identified the risks.

continued . . .

The risks to Francesca if she followed her wishes were as follows.

• *Health risks if her blood pressure was not monitored.*
• *Risks to her emotional well-being if she did not have the opportunity to consider the full implications of giving up her baby.*

The risks to the unborn baby were the following.

• *Unknown health risks – these could not be fully assessed because of the lack of antenatal care.*
• *The emotional risks of not being wanted by her mother.*

We decided to talk with Francesca in a clear and calm manner, explaining that we would support Francesca in whatever decisions she made but we had a responsibility to ensure she was aware of the potential risks. We did this as best we could during the labour. Afterwards we spent more time with Francesca carefully reassuring her that she could change her mind at any point if she did decide to see or hold or feed the baby. In the event, Francesca agreed to stay in the hospital for one night after the birth and to meet with a social worker to talk about her baby. She did, however, go through with her plan of going home and not seeing the baby.

Activity 12.5   *Critical thinking*

Resolving your ethical dilemma

In relation to the ethical dilemma you identified earlier, use the steps outlined above to identify how you found a resolution.

Reflection in action

The third way in which practising within complexity can be developed is through the use of reflection in action. In Chapter 7 we explored in some depth the notion of reflection on action – thinking through an event after it has occurred. Reflection *in* action involves thinking things through reflectively while also taking part in them. Examples might be reflection during a meeting with a service user, in a case review, or while having a telephone conversation. It is one attribute of a professional midwife that they are able to undertake this complex activity

Reflection in action shares many features of other reflective activity.

• It builds on and develops critical thinking.
• It requires a deep approach to learning.
• It explores beneath the surface and so involves challenge, doubt, uncertainty and contra-dictions.
• It uses experiences and feelings as resources to assist in developing an understanding of what is going on.
• It thinks about things from different perspectives.
• It is aided by understanding and self-awareness of how you grasp and deal with things.

However, it is more challenging than reflection on action because it requires all this while you are in the middle of an interaction, rather than in the luxurious position of being able to reflect after the event. So it requires clear, swift and multi-faceted thinking while also being engaged in a conversation or discussion, often in difficult circumstances. The purpose of reflection in action is to be able to understand what is going on at different levels of the interaction, while also being a participant. It should enable a midwife to appreciate if, why and how their approach needs to change – and to be able to respond in a different way. Developing these skills can be helped by:

- building your reflective skills and self-awareness through reflection on action;
- good preparation for interactions, where possible, so you go about your work with a clear mind and open to the unexpected;
- a sound appreciation of theories of human relations such as transference, counter transference, projection and defence mechanisms;
- flexibility in your style – being able to shift your approach in response to your developing understanding of events and processes.

Research summary

In Redmond's (2006) study the students gave their thoughts on reflection in action (p121):

Watch it, realise what's happening and do something about it.

You have to stop yourself and think. You suddenly listen to what you are saying . . . you catch yourself . . . but once you can see what's happening you can be different.

Case study: Linda working with Anya

Linda was supporting Anya in the first stage of an induced labour. The induction, at 38 weeks, was for intra-uterine growth restriction, complicated by Anya being a drug user. Although Anya was on a methadone regime, the medical and social work team involved in her care had concerns that she was also still using heroin or some other drugs. Linda had worked hard to establish a relationship with Anya and her mother Barbara, who was also present, but had found it difficult to cope with Anya insisting on leaving the delivery suite almost every hour in order to smoke. Linda had explained about the necessity of continuous monitoring because of the need to observe the effects of syntocinon and labour on a very small baby, but Anya could not seem to take this seriously. Linda had sought the support of her mentor and a senior registrar, but it seemed that no one could convince Anya of the riskiness of her behaviour.

Linda felt really angry and frustrated with Anya – she could feel these strong feelings welling up inside her. She could not understand why Anya was putting her baby at risk and strongly suspected that Anya could be using the 'fag break' to use other drugs. Turning off and on the syntocinon was also delaying the induction process, but Anya could not see that her behaviour was contributing to this. Despite her strong feelings of annoyance and irritation with Anya – she felt like shouting at her - Linda recognised the risks in displaying her frustration to

continued . . .

Anya. She had to think hard to work out the most helpful plan possible to ensure maximum safety and to continue a working relationship with Anya.

Linda tried to visualise the gap between her and Anya as a chasm and remembered the concept of 'the bridge' that a previous mentor had introduced her to. Her mentor had explained how it was her responsibility as a midwife to always try to build a bridge over the gulf between her and the woman by finding the most helpful way of communicating, thus ensuring it was as easy as possible for the woman to accept guidance and help. Linda kept this image in her head, tried to set her frustration on one side and managed to stay alongside Anya.

Although Linda could not convince Anya to accept the plan of care for her safety and that of her baby, she felt reassured that she had been able to recognise her own very strong feelings and manage them to ensure that her care was the best it could be in difficult circumstances. Afterwards Linda was able to recognise how important it had been to be aware of and acknowledge to herself these strong feelings about Anya in order to ensure that they could be managed in the interests of good practice.

Activity 12.6   *Reflection*

Using reflection in action

Think of an example from your own practice of using reflection in action. Consider how you used reflection in action to support the care required by your client, being guided by the case study of Linda's experience. To complete the process, evaluate your ability to reflect in action and consider how you will continue to apply this principle to other areas of your practice.

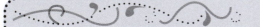

Chapter summary

In this chapter we have explored the complexity and uncertainty of midwifery practice. Appreciating the reasons, context and building on the skills covered in earlier chapters, we have considered three approaches to support constructively working in this context: working in 'secure unknowingness'; using thinking skills to resolve ethical dilemmas; and reflection in action. It should be apparent that taking an active and a deep approach to learning will be required for you to be able to grow and develop to this point. Using these approaches together should enable you to be a professional with reasoning, emotion and intelligence who can react reflectively, recognise many viewpoints and complexities, use a range of skills and knowledge creatively from diverse sources, create knowledge and transfer it to other contexts. This should assist you in making wise decisions in the uncertain conditions of midwifery practice.

Further reading

The following books deal in more depth with ethical dilemmas.

Foster, I and Lasser, J (2011) *Professional ethics in midwifery practice*. London: Jones and Bartlett.

Griffith, R, Tengnah, C A and Patel, C (2010) *Law and professional issues in midwifery*. London: Learning Matters/Sage.

Conclusion

Studying for a degree in midwifery can be exciting, rewarding and challenging. Sometimes the difficulties that students face can overwhelm and obscure the stimulation and thrill of learning. This book arose from our observations that students need support and guidance with developing specific academic skills within the context of studying for midwifery. Without this it can be difficult for students to make progress and maximise their opportunities for personal and professional development. If the book has been a support to you during your degree studies and helped you better to appreciate effective academic study, then it will have achieved its aim.

Having reached this part of the book you will be nearing the end of your midwifery degree. Depending on your mode of study, this might have taken you three or four years and you will be close to qualifying as a midwife. During this time you will have been through many significant learning experiences, both during your time at university and on placement. When you reflect back on this period of your life you will no doubt recall good times and hard times, highs and lows, frustration and joy, pleasure and pain. Take the time to consider how you have changed during your course both personally and professionally. You might find it particularly useful to identify how you have developed as a learner. This understanding will be valuable as you join the profession of midwifery where you will begin a new phase of learning. One theme of the book has been the complexity of midwifery practice and hence the need for practitioners to incorporate different perspectives and think clearly, analytically and reflectively. These skills should equip you to continue to grow and develop in your midwifery career. We wish you well as you enter the profession of midwifery.

Glossary

academic assertiveness   personal confidence as a learner that enables students to manage the challenges of learning and develop their own thinking and voice.

analysis   examining in detail the different aspects and component parts of an issue; considering it from a range of perspectives.

approaches to learning   the disposition towards, or way of going about, learning.

concept   a mental representation; an abstract idea.

continuing professional development   learning and professional development that takes place after you have achieved a social work qualification.

critical friend   someone in your family, social or student network who will read your work, give honest feedback and be prepared to challenge you.

critical thinking   a questioning stance that aims for a deep understanding, taking into account the construction of ideas and their relationship, challenging assumptions and considering alternative perspectives.

dissertation   an extended piece of written work; exploring a student's selected topic by drawing on theory and research; often the final assessed part of an undergraduate programme.

deep learning   learning that engages in a meaningful and reflective way with the issues being studied.

ethics   general principles or statements that guide professional behaviour.

evaluation   identifying and weighing up the strengths and limitations of an issue.

metacognition   the recognition of your own knowledge and processes of knowing and learning.

Personal Development Plan   a reflective record of your needs, progress and achievements as a learner.

plagiarism   taking the work of another person or people and using it as if it were your own; not acknowledging the source of your information or inspiration.

principle   fundamental truth or proposition on which action is based.

qualitative   concerned with experiences, opinions, feelings, behaviour and attitudes.

quantitative   concerned with numbers and statistics.

reflection   the purposeful process of consideration and reconsideration of any aspect of learning – knowledge, theory and experiences.

research   the systematic investigation into, and study of, sources of material in order to establish facts and reach new conclusions.

second-order reflection   reconsidering a piece of reflective writing in order to reflect again and develop new insights.

self-efficacy   being able to take ownership of your learning and its challenges.

strategic learning   learning that uses specific strategies to achieve the desired outcome rather than fully engaging in the process.

surface learning   learning that is superficial – does not fully engage with the deeper meaning and relationships of the issues being studied.

synthesis   bringing together different contributions to understanding a topic in order to appreciate it in depth and understand it in a new way.

theory   a set of related ideas that helps to explain or make sense of an issue.

values   a collection of beliefs or principles about what is important.

References

Abbott, P, Wallace, C and Tyler, M (2005) *An introduction to sociology: feminist perspectives*. London: Routledge.

Ainsworth, A (2013) Changing childbirth practices – an impossible job? What can we learn from the world of organisational change? *Midwifery Matters*, 136: 8–10.

Alcock, P (2003) *Social policy in Britain* (2nd edition). Basingstoke: Palgrave Macmillan.

Alcock, C, Daly, G and Griggs, E (2008) *Introducing social policy* (2nd edition). Harlow: Pearson.

Andersson, O, Hellström-Westas, L, Andersson, D and Domellöf, M (2011) Effect of delayed versus early umbilical cord clamping on neonatal outcomes and iron status at 4 months: a randomised controlled trial. *British Medical Journal*, 343: d7157.

Armstrong, N (2008) Role modelling in the clinical workplace. *British Journal of Midwifery*, 16 (9): 596–603.

Bach, S and Grant, A (2011) *Communication and interpersonal skills in nursing* (2nd edition). Exeter: Learning Matters.

Barkley, A (2011) Ideals, expectations and reality: challenges for student midwives. *British Journal of Midwifery*, 19 (4): 259–64.

Barnett, R (1994) *The limits of competence: knowledge, higher education and society*. Buckingham: Open University Press.

Baxter, J and Pride, J (2008) Should midwives wear uniforms? Let's ask the women. *British Journal of Midwifery*, 16 (8): 523–26.

Begley, C M, Gyte, G M L, Devane, D, McGuire, W and Weeks, A (2011) Active versus expectant management for women in the third stage of labour. *Cochrane Database of Systematic Reviews*, Issue 11. Art. No. CD007412.

Biggs, J B (2003) *Teaching for quality learning at university* (2nd edition). Buckingham: Open University Press/Society for Research into Higher Education.

Biggs, J and Tang, C (2011) *Teaching for quality learning at university* (4th edition). Maidenhead: Open University Press/McGraw Hill.

BirthChoice UK (2013) *Where to have your baby*. Available at: www.birthchoiceuk.com/BirthChoiceUK Frame.htm.

Bolton, G (2010) *Reflective practice: writing and professional development*. London: Sage.

Boud, D and Solomon, N (eds) (2001) *Work-based learning: a new higher education?* Maidenhead: Open University Press.

Boud, D, Keogh, R and Walker, D (1985) *Reflection: turning experience into learning*. London: Kogan Page.

Breheny, M and Stephens, C (2010) Youth or disadvantage? The construction of teenage mothers in medical journals. *Culture, Health and Sexuality*, 12 (3): 307–22.

Brocklehurst, P, Hardy, P, Hollowell, J, Linsell, L, Macfarlane, A, McCourt, C et al. (Birthplace in England Collaborative Group) (2011) Perinatal and maternal outcomes by planned place of birth for healthy women with low risk pregnancies: the Birthplace in England national prospective cohort study. *British Medical Journal*, 343: d7400: 1–13.

Bryar, R and Sinclair, M (eds) (2011) *Theory for midwifery practice* (2nd edition). Basingstoke: Palgrave Macmillan.

Burke, D (2007) How students use feedback. Paper presented at the Association for Learning and Development in Higher Education Symposium, 12 April.

Campbell, D (2012) Health Bill explained. *Guardian*, 15 March.

Carolan, M and Hodnett, E (2007) 'With woman' philosophy: examining the evidence, answering the questions. *Nursing Inquiry*, 14 (2): 140–52.

Carr, W (1995) *For education: towards critical educational enquiry*. Buckingham: Open University Press.

Chan, V. (2001) Readiness for learner autonomy: what do our learners tell us? *Teaching in Higher Education*, 6 (4): 505–18.

Chief Nursing Officers of England, Northern Ireland, Scotland and Wales (2010) *Midwifery 2020: delivering expectations*. London: Department of Health.

Clare, B (2007) Promoting deep learning: a teaching, learning and assessment endeavour. *Social Work Education*, 26 (5): 433–46.

Clarke, E (2011) One hundred days as a direct entry student midwife: a personal account. *British Journal of Midwifery*, 19 (9): 600–02.

Clarke, J and Newman, J (1997) *The managerial state*. London: Sage.

Cluett, E R and Bluff, R (eds) (2006) *Principles and practice of midwifery research* (2nd edition). Edinburgh: Elsevier.

CEMACE (2011) Saving mothers' lives: reviewing maternal deaths to make motherhood safer: 2006–2008. The Eighth Report of the Confidential Enquiries into Maternal Deaths in the United Kingdom. *British Journal of Obstetrics and Gynaecology*, 118 (S1): 1–203. First published online, March 2011.

Coffield, F (2009) *All you ever wanted to know about learning and teaching but were too cool to ask*. London: Learning and Skills Network.

Collington, V and Hunt, S (2006) Reflection in midwifery education and practice: an exploratory analysis. *Evidence Based Midwifery*, 4 (3): 76–82.

Common, L (2007) Studying: ways to survive and thrive. *Midwives Magazine*, Nov/Dec.

Cottrell, S (2011) *Critical thinking skills* (2nd edition). Basingstoke: Palgrave Macmillan.

Cottrell, S (2013) *The study skills handbook* (4th edition). Basingstoke: Palgrave Macmillan.

CQC (Care Quality Commission) (2010) *Maternity services survey 2010*. Available at: www.cqc.org.uk/public/reports-surveys-and-reviews/surveys/maternity-services-survey-2010.

Cree, V and Macauley, C (eds) (2000) *Transfer of learning in professional and vocational education*. London: Routledge.

Cronk, M and Jowitt, M (1997) *Radical midwifery*. London: ARM.

Dearnley, C and Matthew, B (2007) Factors that contribute to undergraduate success. *Teaching in Higher Education*, 12 (3): 377–91.

DCSF (Department for Children, Schools and Families) (2010) *Common assessment framework*. London: DCSF.

DfE (Department for Education) (2013) *Working together to safeguard children*. London: DfE.

Derounian, J (2011) Shall we dance? The importance of staff–student relationships to undergraduate dissertation preparation. *Active Learning in Higher Education*, 12: 91.

DH (Department of Health) (2000) *Framework for assessment of children in need and their families*. London: DH.

DH (2004) *The NHS Knowledge and Skills Framework (NHS KSF) and the development review process.* London: DH.

DH (2007) *Maternity matters: choice, access and continuity of care in a safe service.* London: Department of Health.

DH (2010) *Midwifery 2020: delivering expectations.* London: Department of Health.

DH (2012) *Breastfeeding initiation and prevalence at 6–8 weeks, Quarter 2, 2011/12.* London: Department of Health. Available at: www.dh.gov.uk/en/Publicationsandstatistics/Publications/PublicationsStatistics/DH_130857 (Crown Copyright).

DHSS (Department of Health and Social Security) (1972) *Report of the Committee of Nursing (Briggs Report).* London: HMSO (Cmnd 5115).

Dobash, R and Dobash, R (1980) *Violence against wives: a case against the patriarchy.* Shepton Mallet: Open Books.

Dow, A (2012) Simulation-based learning: a case study, part 3. *British Journal of Midwifery,* 20 (9): 654–58.

Downe, S (2012) Skilled help from the heart: the story of a midwifery research programme. *Evidence Based Midwifery,* 10 (1): 4–9.

Duffy, A (2007) A concept analysis of reflective practice: determining its value to nurses. *British Journal of Nursing,* 16 (22): 1400–07.

Dunn, D M (2010) *Twelve babies on a bike: diary of a pupil midwife.* London: Orion.

Edwards, R (1993) *Mature women students: separating or connecting family and education.* London: Routledge.

Ellis, P (2010) *Understanding research for nursing students.* Exeter: Learning Matters.

Entwistle, N, McCune, V and Walker, P (2001) Conceptions, styles and approaches within higher education: analytical abstractions and everyday experiences. In Sternberg, R and Zhang, L (eds) (2001) *Perspectives on thinking, learning and cognitive styles.* London: Lawrence Erlbaum Associates.

Eraut, M (1994) *Developing professional knowledge and competence.* London: Falmer Press.

Fonteyn, M E and Cahill, M (1998) The use of clinical logs to improve nursing students' metacognition: a pilot study. *Journal of Advanced Nursing,* 28 (1): 149–54.

Foster, I R and Lasser, J (2010) *Professional ethics in midwifery practice.* Burlington, MA: Jones and Bartlett.

Francis, R (2013) *Report of the Mid Staffordshire NHS Foundation Trust Public Inquiry.* London: Stationery Office.

Freire, P (1972) *Pedagogy of the oppressed.* London: Penguin.

Gardosi J, Madurasinghe V, Williams S, Malik, A and Francis, A (2013) Maternal and fetal risk factors for stillbirth: population based study. *British Medical Journal,* 346: f108: 1–14.

Ghate, D and Hazel, N (2003) *Parenting in poor environments.* London: Jessica Kingsley.

Gibbs, G (1981) *Teaching students to learn.* Milton Keynes: Open University Press.

Gibbs, G (2010) *Dimensions of quality.* York: Higher Education Academy.

Gimenez, J (2012) Disciplinary epistemologies, generic attributes and undergraduate academic writing in nursing and midwifery. *Higher Education,* 63: 401–19.

Gordon, J and Cooper B (2010) Talking knowledge – practising knowledge: a critical best practice approach to how social workers use and understand knowledge in practice. *Practice,* 22 (4): 245–57.

Gross, R (2010) *Psychology: the science of mind and behaviour.* London: Hodder Education.

Hannah, M E, Hannah, W J, Hewson, S, Hodnett, E, Saigal, S, Willan, A. for the Term Breech Trial Collaborative Group (2000) Planned caesarean section versus planned vaginal birth for breech presentation at term: a randomised multicentre trial. *The Lancet (*356) 1375–83.

Hannigan, B and Burnard, P (2001) Preparing and writing an undergraduate dissertation. *Nurse Education in Practice*, 1: 175–180.

Hodnett E D, Downe S and Walsh, D (2012) Alternative versus conventional institutional settings for birth. *Cochrane Database of Systematic Reviews* 2012, Issue 8. Art. No: CD000012. DOI: 10.1002/14651858. CD000012.pub4.

Horwath, J (ed.) (2002) *The child's world: assessing children in need.* London: Jessica Kingsley.

Howard, D (2002) Changes in nursing students' out of college relationships arising from the Diploma of Higher Education in Nursing. *Active Learning in Higher Education*, 3 (1): 68–87.

Howarth, A (1999) The portfolio as an assessment tool in midwifery education. *British Journal of Midwifery*, 7 (5): 327–29.

Howatson-Jones, L (2013) *Reflective practice in nursing* (2nd edition). Exeter: Learning Matters.

Howe, D (2001) Attachment. In Horwath, J (ed.) *The child's world: assessing children in need.* London: Jessica Kingsley, pp194–206.

Howe, D (2007) Relating theory to practice. In Davies, M (ed.) *Companion to social work* (3rd edition). Oxford: Blackwell.

Hunt, S (2004) *Poverty, pregnancy and the healthcare professional.* Edinburgh: Books for Midwives.

Jackson, N (2004) Developing the concept of metalearning. *Innovations in Education and Teaching International*, 41 (4): 391–403.

Johns, C (2009) *Becoming a reflective practitioner.* Oxford: Wiley Blackwell.

Jones, L, Othman, M, Dowswell, T, Alfirevic, Z, Gates, S, Newburn, M, Jordan, S, Lavender, T and Neilson, J P (2012) Pain management for women in labour: an overview of systematic reviews. *Cochrane Database of Systematic Reviews 2012*, Issue 3, Art. No. CD009234. DOI: 10.1002/14651858.CD009234.pub2.

Jowitt, M (2013) The new vision for maternity care. *Midwifery Matters*, 136: 2.

Kerrigan, A and Houghton, G (2010) Including marginalised groups in maternity research: the challenges for midwives. *Evidence Based Midwifery*, 8 (1): 4–7.

Kingdon, C (2008) *Sociology for midwives.* London: Quay Books.

Kirkham, M (ed.) (2010) *The midwife–mother relationship* (2nd edition) Basingstoke: Palgrave Macmillan.

Kirkham, M (2013) Modern birth: processes and fears. *Midwifery Matters*, 1: 36.

Kolcaba, K Y (1994) A theory of holistic comfort for nursing. *Journal of Advanced Nursing*, 19 (6): 1178–84.

Laming, Lord H (2003) *The Victoria Climbié inquiry report.* CM 5730. London: The Stationery Office. Crown copyright.

Leap, N (1996) Persuading women to give birth at home – or offering real choice? *British Journal of Midwifery*, 4 (10): 536–38.

Leap, N and Anderson, P (2008) The role of pain in normal birth and the empowerment of women. In Downe, S (ed.) *Normal childbirth: evidence and debate* (2nd edition). London: Churchill Livingstone.

Levett-Jones T L (2007) Facilitating reflective practice and self-assessment of competence through the use of narratives. *Nurse Education in Practice*, 7: 112–19.

Lewis, P (2011) A journey of discovery and delight. *MIDIRS*, 2 (8): 4.

Lewis, P (2013) A house of cards: the futility of a service that fails to listen. *British Journal of Midwifery*, 21 (3): 158.

Lipp, A (2010) Conceding and concealing judgement in termination of pregnancy; a grounded theory study. *Journal of Research in Nursing*, 15 (4): 365–78.

Lishman, J (ed.) (2007) *Handbook for practice learning in social work and social care* (2nd edition). London: Jessica Kingsley.

Lister, P G (2000) Mature students and transfer of learning. In Cree, V and Macauley, C (eds) *Transfer of learning in professional and vocational education*. London: Routledge.

Lyons, F and Bennett, M (2001) Setting the standards: judging levels of achievement. In Boud, D and Solomon, N (eds) *Work-based learning. A new higher education?* Buckingham: Open University Press.

Macaulay, C (2000) Transfer of learning. In Cree, V and Macaulay, C (eds) *Transfer of learning in professional and vocational education*. London: Routledge.

Madden, E, Sinclair, M and Wright, M. (2011) Teamwork in obstetric emergencies. *Evidence Based Midwifery*, 9 (3): 95–101.

Mander, R (2011) Who chooses the choices? *Modern Midwife*, 3 (1): 23–25.

Marshall, D and Case, J (2005) Approaches to learning research in higher education: a response to haggis. *British Educational Research Journal*, 31 (2): 257–67.

McCann, L and Saunders, G (2008) Improving students' perceptions of assessment feedback. Available at: www.swap.ac.uk/resources/publs/casestudies/saunders.html.

McCowan, L M E, Dekker, G A, Chan, E, Stewart, A, Chappell, L C, Hunter, M, Moss-Morris, R and North, R A (2009) Spontaneous preterm birth and small for gestational age infants in women who stop smoking early in pregnancy: prospective cohort study. *British Medical Journal*, 338: b1081

McCutcheon, R and Brown, D (2012) A qualitative exploration of women's experiences of giving birth at home. *Evidence Based Midwifery*, 10 (1): 23–28.

McInnes, R J and McIntosh C (2012) What future for midwifery? *Nurse Education in Practice*, 12: 297–300.

McMillan, W J (2010) 'Your thrust is to understand' – how academically successful students learn. *Teaching in Higher Education*, 15 (1): 1–13.

Mezirow, J (1981) A critical theory of adult learning and education. *Adult Education*, 32 (1): 3–24.

Miles, S (2008) Make or break: the importance of good mentorship. *British Journal of Midwifery* 16 (1): 704–71.

Moon, J (2004) *A handbook of reflective and experiential learning*. London: Routledge Falmer.

Moon, J (2005) *We seek it here . . . a new perspective on the elusive activity of critical thinking: a theoretical and practical approach*. Bristol: ESCalate.

Moon, J (2008) *Critical thinking: an exploration of theory and practice*. London: Routledge.

Newburn, M (2012) The best of both worlds: parents' motivations for using an alongside birth centre from an ethnographic study. *Midwifery*, 28 (1): 61–66.

NHSIC (NHS Information Centre) (2013) *NHS Maternity Statistics – England, 2010–2011*. Available at: www.ic.nhs.uk/pubs/maternity1011.

NICE (National Institute for Health and Clinical [Care] Excellence) (2005) *Breastfeeding for longer – what works? Systematic review summary*. London: NICE.

NICE (2008) *Antenatal care: full guidelines*. London: NICE. Available at: http://guidance.nice.org.uk/CG62/.

NMC (Nursing and Midwifery Council) (2008) *The code: standards of conduct, performance and ethics for nurses and midwives*. Available to download from www.nmc-uk.org.

NMC (2009) *Standards for pre-registration midwifery education*. London: NMC.

NMC (2010) *Guidance on professional conduct for nursing and midwifery students*. Available to download from www.nmc-uk.org.

NMC (2011a) *The prep handbook*. London: NMC.

NMC (2011b) Guidance on post-registration education and practice. Available to download from www.nmc-uk.org.

NMC (2012) *Midwives rules and standards*. Available to download from www.nmc-uk.org.

NMC (2013a) *The quality assurance framework: for nursing and midwifery education and local supervising authorities for midwifery*. Available to download from www.nmc-uk.org .

NMC (2013b) *Guidance on professional conduct for nursing and midwifery students*. London: NMC. Available to download from www.nmc-uk.org.

NPEU (National Perinatal and Epidemiology Unit) (2007) *Recorded delivery: a national survey of women's experiences of maternity care*. Oxford: NPEU.

NPEU (2010) *Delivered with care: a national survey of women's experience of maternity care*. Oxford: NPEU. Available at: www.npeu.ox.ac.uk/files/downloads/reports/Maternity-Survey-Report-2010.pdf.

Nyman, V, Downe, S and Berg, M (2011) Waiting for permission to enter the labour ward world: first-time parents' experiences of the first encounter on a labour ward. *Sexual & Reproductive Healthcare*, 2: 129–34.

Oakley, A (2005) *The Ann Oakley reader*. Bristol: Polity Press.

O'Connell, R and Downe, S (2009) A metasynthesis of midwives' experience of hospital practice in publicly funded settings: compliance, resistance and authenticity *Health*, 13 (6): 589–609.

Office for National Statistics (2013) *Statistical Bulletin: Live Births in England and Wales by Characteristics of Mother 1. 2011*. London: The Stationery Office.

Oliver, M and Sapey, B (2006) *Social work with disabled people*. Basingstoke: Macmillan.

Olsen, O and Clausen, J A (2012) Planned hospital birth versus planned home birth. *Cochrane Database of Systematic Reviews*, Issue 9. Art. no. CD000352. DOI: 10.1002/14651858.CD000352.pub2.

Page. L (2013) Journeys of the RCM president: exploring midwifery practice. *British Journal of Midwifery*, 21 (1): 6.

Paradice, R (2002) *Psychology for midwives*. London: Quay Books.

Parker, J (2010) *Effective practice learning in social work* (2nd edition). Exeter: Learning Matters.

Pierson, J (2002) *Tackling social exclusion*. London: Routledge.

Price, B and Harrington, A (2010) *Critical thinking and writing for nursing students*. Exeter: Learning Matters/Sage.

QAA (Quality Assurance Agency for Higher Education) (2008) *The framework for higher education qualifications in England, Wales and Northern Ireland*. Gloucester: QAA. Available to download from www.qaa.ac.uk.

Race, P (2010) *Making learning happen* (2nd edition). London: Sage.

Raynor, M and England, C (2010) *Psychology for midwives*. Maidenhead: Open University Press.

RCM (Royal College of Midwives) (2008a) *Women centred care: position statement*. London: RCM.

RCM (2008b) *Supporting women in labour: midwifery practice guidelines*. London: RCM.

RCM (2011a) The Royal College of Midwives Survey of Midwives' current thinking about home birth. London: RCM. Available at: www.rcm.org.uk/EasySiteWeb/GatewayLink.aspx?alId=185762.

RCM (2011b) *State of maternity services report 2011*. London: RCM

RCOG (Royal College of Obstetricians and Gynaecologists) (2011) *High quality women's health care*. London: RCOG. Available at: www.rcog.org.uk/high-quality-womens-health-care.

Redmond, B (2006) *Reflection in action*. Aldershot: Ashgate.

Redshaw, M (2006) First relationships and the growth of love. In Page, L A and McCandlish, R (eds) *The new midwifery* (2nd edition). Edinburgh: Churchill Livingstone.

Redshaw, M and Heikka, K (2010) *Delivered with care: a national survey of women's experience of maternity care*. Oxford: NPEU.

Rees, C (2011) *Introduction to research for midwives* (3rd edition). London: Churchill Livingstone.

Reisz, M (2008) Hits and misses. *Times Higher Education*, 5–12 June, 1848: 32.

Robinson, L. (2008) *Psychology for social workers* (2nd edition). London: Routledge.

Rogers, C R (1961) *On becoming a person*. Boston: Houghton Mifflin.

Ross, T (2012) *A survival guide for health research methods*. Maidenhead: Open University Press.

Rowe, R, Fitzpatrick, R, Hollowell, J and Kurinczuk, J (2012a) Transfers of women planning birth in midwifery units: data from the birthplace prospective cohort study. *BJOG: An International Journal of Obstetrics & Gynaecology*, 119: 1081–90.

Rowe, R, Kurinczuk, J J, Locock, L and Fitzpatrick, R. (2012b) Women's experience of transfer from midwifery unit to hospital obstetric unit during labour: a qualitative interview study. *BMC Pregnancy Childbirth*, doi: 10.1186/1471–2393–12–129.

Salkind, N J (2011) *Statistics for people who (think they) hate statistics*. London: Sage.

Schön, D A (1983) *The reflective practitioner: how professionals think in action*. New York: Basic Books.

Schroeder, S, Petrou, S, Patel, N, Hollowell, J, Puddicombe, D, Redshaw, M and Brocklehurst, P (2012) Cost effectiveness of alternative planned places of birth in woman at low risk of complications: evidence from the Birthplace in England national prospective cohort study. *British Medical Journal*, 344, e2292: 1–13.

Schuiling, K D, Sampselle, C and Kolcaba, K (2011) Exploring the presence of comfort within the context of childbirth. In Bryar, R and Sinclair, M (eds) *Theory for midwifery practice* (2nd edition). Basingstoke: Palgrave Macmillan.

Secker, J. (1993) *From theory to practice in social work*. Aldershot: Avebury.

Shardlow, S (2007) The social policy context of practice learning. In Lishman, J (ed.) *Handbook for practice learning in social work and social care*. London: Jessica Kingsley.

Singh D and Newburn, M (2000) *Access to maternity information and support: the experiences of women before and after giving birth*. London: National Childbirth Trust.

Stapleton, H, Kirkham, M, Thomas, G and Curtis, P (2002) Language used in antenatal consultations. *British Journal of Midwifery*, 10 (5): 273–77.

Steen, M and Roberts, T (2011) *The handbook of midwifery research*. Oxford: Wiley.

Stephenson, J. (2001) Ensuring a holistic approach to work-based learning. In Boud, D and Solomon, N (eds) *Work-based learning. A new higher education?* Buckingham: Open University Press.

Stuart, C C (2010) The reflective journeys of a midwife tutor and her students. *Reflective Practice*, 2 (2): 171–84.

Symon, A and Lee, J (2003) Including men in antenatal education: evaluating innovative practice. *Evidence Based Midwifery*, 1 (1).

Taylor, B (2010) *Reflective practice for healthcare professionals*. Maidenhead: McGraw Hill.

Taylor, C and White, S (2000) *Practising reflexivity in health and welfare*. Buckingham: University Press.

Tew, M (1998) *Safer childbirth? A critical history of maternity care*. London: Free Association Books.

Thompson, N (2000) *Theory and practice in human services*. Maidenhead: Open University Press.

Thompson, N (2006) *Anti-discriminatory practice*. Basingstoke: Palgrave Macmillan.

Thorpe, M. (2000) Encouraging students to reflect as part of the assignment process. *Active Learning in Higher Education*, 1 (1): 79–92.

Todd, M J, Bannister, P and Clegg, S (2004) Independent inquiry and the undergraduate dissertation: perceptions and experiences of final year social science students. *Assessment and Evaluation in Higher Education*, 29 (3): 335–55.

Todd, M J, Smith, K and Bannister, P (2006) Supervising a social science undergraduate dissertation: staff experiences and perceptions. *Teaching in Higher Education*, 11 (2): 161–73.

Walker, H (2011) *Studying for your social work degree*. Exeter: Learning Matters.

Walsh, D (2007) *Evidence-based care for normal labour and birth*. London: Routledge.

Watson, F, Burrows, H and Player, C (2002) *Integrating theory and practice in social work education*. London and New York: Jessica Kingsley.

Way, S (2011) The combined use of diaries and interviewing for the collection of data in midwifery research. *Evidence Based Midwifery*, 9 (2): 66–70.

Wickham, S (2006) *Appraising research into childbirth*. London: Elsevier.

Williams, F (1989) *Social policy: a critical introduction*. Oxford: Polity Press.

Worth, J (2008) *Call the midwife: a true story of the East End in the 1950s*. London: Phoenix.

Index